A–Z of Dental Nursing

Wendy Paintin

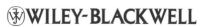

WILEY-BLACKWELL

A John Wiley & Sons, Ltd., Publication

This edition first published 2009
© 2009 by Blackwell Publishing Ltd

Blackwell Publishing was acquired by John Wiley & Sons in February 2007.
Blackwell's publishing programme has been merged with Wiley's global
Scientific, Technical, and Medical business to form Wiley-Blackwell.

Registered office
John Wiley & Sons Ltd, The Atrium, Southern Gate, Chichester, West Sussex,
PO19 8SQ, United Kingdom

Editorial offices
9600 Garsington Road, Oxford, OX4 2DQ, United Kingdom
2121 State Avenue, Ames, Iowa 50014-8300, USA

For details of our global editorial offices, for customer services and for
information about how to apply for permission to reuse the copyright
material in this book please see our website at www.wiley.com/
wiley-blackwell.

Library of Congress Cataloging-in-Publication Data

Paintin, Wendy.
  A–Z of dental nursing / Wendy Paintin.
      p. ; cm.
  ISBN 978-1-4051-7908-9 (pbk. : alk. paper)   1. Dentistry–Dictionaries.
2. Dental auxiliary personnel–Handbooks, manuals, etc.   I. Title.
II. Title: A to Z of dental nursing.
  [DNLM: 1. Dentistry–Handbooks.   2. Dentistry–
Terminology–English.   3. Dental Assistants–Handbooks.   4. Dental
Assistants–Terminology–English. WU 49 P148a 2009]
  RK27.P35 2009
  617.6003–dc22

                                                            2008023779

A catalogue record for this book is available from the British Library.

Set in 9 on 11 pt Palatino by SNP Best-set Typesetter Ltd., Hong Kong
Printed in Singapore by Fabulous Printers Pte Ltd

1   2009

Contents

Introduction

This book is for dental nurses at all stages of their career development, be they trainee, just qualified or experienced. The book functions as an aide memoire to practising dental nurses, as an essential reference book for trainee nurses and as a teaching aid for assessors and tutors in further education.

The A–Z can be used as a learning/revision aid and reference book providing concise, accurate and clear-cut definitions of common words, terms, names and phrases associated with the occupation. Typical examples of the broad subjects included are names of instruments, medical terminology, anatomy, physiology, cross infection and surgery equipment, as well as all aspects of patient management.

The *A–Z of Dental Nursing* consists of data that exists in various formats within existing, separate publications, but gathers this together, centralises, and demystifies it, while augmenting it with years of on the job experience. This approach, coupled with the pocket-sized format, results in a single, reliable source of relevant, detailed knowledge in a user-friendly layout. Each word has a keyword reference that can be used as a guide when researching the topic in associated materials.

An important distinctive feature of this book is its structure; it provides the essential information, broken down into bite size chunks and presented in a user-friendly format that does not require the material to be read from cover to cover in order to achieve an understanding of the subject.

The A–Z is intended to become a dental nurse's 'best friend'; a companion and guide that, through regular use, you will come to rely on.

The A–Z also includes common abbreviations used in note taking/writing, charting, information about career paths in the occupation, details of professional bodies, related training courses and publications and useful websites.

About the Author

Wendy Paintin is a qualified Dental Nurse with fifteen years' experience in the profession, including general dentistry, private dentistry, cosmetic dentistry, community dental services and emergency access centres, hospitals/minor oral surgery as well as training, teaching and assessing nurses who are working towards achieving an NVQ level 3 qualification. She is also a member of the health and safety committee for the British Association of Dental Nurses.

Part 1

A–Z of Terms and Concepts

Abdomen

What non-medics might refer to as their belly; strictly speaking, it's the cavity between the chest and pelvis, containing the stomach, intestines, kidneys, liver, pancreas and spleen.

Keywords: Anatomy/digestion

Abrasion

Damage affecting certain cervical surfaces, caused by pressing too hard when brushing the teeth.

Keyword: Dental disorders

Abscess

Localised collection of pus. An abscess may be periapical or periodontal depending on its position. Caused by bacteria invading the pulp and spreading to the surrounding tissues.

Keyword: Pathology

Abutment

Used during dental implant placement. Available in different diameters and heights. They're used as part of the soft tissue management process. The temporary abutment is attached to the implant and will be replaced by a permanent one once the implant has bonded with the bony tissue and healing has completed. Later the super-structure is placed on the permanent abutment.

Keyword: Implants

Abutment depth gauge

Part of a dental implant kit, this instrument is used to measure in millimetres the mucosal height over the implant level.

Keyword: Implants

Aciclovir
An antiviral drug prescribed for treating cold sores on the lips and mouth ulcers caused by the herpes virus.

Keyword: Drugs

Acid etching
Gel or liquid applied to the tooth surface to gain retention for the filling material, allowing the material to bond directly to the enamel.

Keyword: Composite filling

Acrylic
Heat-cured acrylic is used for making dentures or orthodontic appliances. Cold-cured acrylic is used for making of temporary crowns and denture repairs. Polymer powder and monomer liquid, when mixed together, form a plastic mass which can be heated in an oven (heat cured) or set at room temperature by assigning a catalyst (cold self cured).

Keyword: Dentures

Acquired immune deficiency syndrome (AIDS)
Deficiency of the immune system due to infection with HIV (human immunodeficiency virus). The body's defence mechanism is destroyed resulting in an inability to resist infection. HIV is a blood-borne virus, therefore care must be taken with infected blood, needles and instruments. No cure or vaccine is available.

Keywords: Pathology/infection control

Acute lateral periodontal abscess
This infection occurs on a vital tooth at the side of the root.

Keyword: Pathology

Acute necrotising ulcerative gingivitis (ANUG)
Usually affects people who already have chronic gingivitis. Symptoms are: pain, halitosis, bright red gums and raised temperature. Stress, smoking, lowered general health and flu can contribute to an attack. Common in people with AIDS, and can be first sign of the virus.

Keyword: Periodontal disease

A

Acute periapical abscess
This infection occurs at the root apex following the death of the pulp.

Keyword: Pathology

Adams crib
Orthodontic appliance used to retain a removable acrylic-based appliance positioned around the first molars and premolars.

Keyword: Orthodontics

Adams pliers
Orthodontics equipment used to adjust the metal components of an orthodontic appliance.

Keyword: Orthodontics

Adhesive bridge
This fixed prosthetic appliance is used primarily on front teeth. The retaining natural teeth have to be prepared but this is minimal, usually just a bit of the surface removed and roughened in order for metal wings to be bonded to them providing retention for the pontic which replaces the missing tooth/teeth. The retaining teeth need to be healthy and have no heavy fillings.

Keyword: Prosthetic

Adrenaline
Haemostatic drug, most common vasoconstrictor used. Results in narrowing of the blood vessels in the immediate vicinity of the injection so that the solution is not carried away too quickly. This lengthens the time of the anaesthetic to allow treatment to be carried out without the patient feeling any pain.

Keyword: Drugs

Advanced life support (ALS)
The next step after basic life support, if the heart has stopped beating. A powerful electric shock to the heart muscle using a defibrillator is the most effective way of restoring heart function.

Keyword: Collapse

A

Air rotor handpiece
Known as a high-speed handpiece. Water is run through it to cool the tooth as it creates heat and friction. A bur is attached to the handpiece and removes old filling and tooth tissues ready for the preparation of a cavity or a prosthetic work.

Keywords: Instruments/restoration

Air turbine handpiece
Uses diamond or tungsten carbide burs to cut the tooth surface, dentine or old fillings.

Keyword: Restorations

Air water syringe
Also know as triple air syringe or 3-in-1. A disposable tip is attached to a connector and the handle provides control tips for air and water or both together.

Keyword: Instruments

Airway
Passage through which air enters and leaves the lungs. Can also be a tube inserted into the mouth of an unconscious person thus preventing the tongue from obstructing breathing.

Keyword: Respiration

Airway obstruction
This is something that is blocking the passage that carries air to the lungs, making breathing difficult and reducing the amount of air inhaled. This can happen in the nose, mouth or throat. The trachea/windpipe can be obstructed by the swallowing of a foreign object becoming stuck in the digestive tract. Asthma, heart attack and many other things can be the cause of airway construction.

Keyword: Medical emergency/first aid

Alginate
Impression material used for dentures, orthodontic appliances, temporary crowns, bridges and veneers. The elasticity of the material gives an accurate impression from undercut areas

without distortion. Prepare the material by mixing the powder and water together with a spatula and bowl.

Keyword: Prosthetic/restorations

Alimentary canal
Tube-like structure which allows the passage of food from the mouth to the anus.

Keyword: Digestion

Allergy
Violent reaction of the immune system caused by a variety of substances. Has various conditions, most common is asthma.

Keyword: Pathology

Aluminium crown forms
Used as a temporary crown on a prepped tooth whilst the permanent crown is being constructed in the laboratory. This protects the tooth and maintains the gum margins. It is usually cemented with temporary cement for easy removal.

Keyword: Restorations

Aluminium spatula
Used to mix dental materials. This particular type will not discolour nor stick to any materials.

Keyword: Instruments

Alveolar abscess
An abscess caused in the alveolar ridge of the jaw by the spread of infection from an adjacent non-vital tooth.

Keyword: Pathology

Alveolar process
Bone cavity or socket supporting each tooth in the jaw.

Keyword: Anatomy

Alveolectomy
Surgical procedure to smooth out uneven bone, usually done prior to making dentures to ensure better fit.

Keyword: Minor oral surgery

A

Amalgam
Permanent filling material consisting of mercury and other powdered alloy, mixed together and used in posterior teeth.

Keyword: Restoration

Amalgamator
This machine vibrates and has a time set according to the size of the amalgam capsule or mix. Some machines can mix other encapsulated materials as well.

Keyword: Restorations

Amalgam capsule
Contains amalgam material and is disposable. Available in different amounts and is mixed using an amalgamator.

Keyword: Restorations

Amalgam carrier
This instrument is pushed into a pot of amalgam and loads small amounts of the material which is then placed in the prepared cavity.

Keyword: Tooth restoration

Amalgam plugger
Removes excess mercury from amalgam by pressing the filling instrument into the cavity where amalgam has been placed.

Keyword: Restoration

Amalgam safe container
Issued to surgeries by a waste management company. The container is air tight and holds foam inserts that contain non-hazardous chemicals that suppress mercury vapours. They are collected by the hazardous waste management company by arrangement.

Keyword: Health and safety

Amalgam separators
There are several types available and their purpose is to reduce the amount of waste amalgam discharged into the sewer. Depend-

ing on the type of separator, they can be fitted either to the chair or service the whole practice.

Keyword: Health and safety

Amalgam waste
Amalgam and mercury waste should be stored in sealed, labelled containers which have mercury suppressing solution or pastes enclosed. These containers will be provided by the waste company upon request. Amalgam filled extracted teeth should be disposed in amalgam waste, but there are containers available for this.

Keyword: Health and safety

Amber shield
Orange in colour and is used to protect eyes from the curing light.

Keyword: Restorations

Ameloblast cell
These cells lie at the amelodentinal junction. They form the enamel before tooth eruption.

Keyword: Anatomy

Amelodental junction
See Amelodentinal junction

Amelodentinal junction
This describes the surface of a tooth where the enamel and the dentine of the crown meet.

Keyword: Anatomy

Amoxicillin
A penicillin-based drug with a wider range of antibacterial action. Taken by mouth to treat a variety of infections.

Keyword: Drugs

Amphotericin
A drug used to treat fungal infections such as denture stomatitis and angular cheilitis. Applied using a gel or taken as a lozenge or pastille.

Keyword: Drugs

Anaemia

Disorder of the blood. The capacity of red blood cells to carry oxygen is below normal or the blood is unable to carry oxygen due to low number of red blood cells. There are different types of this condition and the most common cause is iron deficiency. Anaemia can happen during pregnancy or can occur due to lack of certain vitamins (usually B12) or iron. Symptoms include feeling tired, faint and breathless; a blood test will confirm a diagnosis.

Keyword: Pathology

Anaesthesia

General: Induced by intravenous injection or internally by inhalation to give loss of sensation.

Local: Loss of sensation in a localised area to prevent pain during procedure. Administered by injection.

Keyword: Anaesthesia

Anaesthetic cartridge

Glass or plastic, single use and disposable containing the local anaesthetic solution.

Keyword: Drugs

Analgesia

Meaning loss of pain only. Sensitivity to pressure is still present. Patient is conscious.

Keyword: Drugs

Analgesics

Drugs used to relieve pain administered internally or externally.

Keyword: Drugs

Anaphylactic shock

Serious type of allergy which can result in a severe state of collapse and may be fatal. The reaction is rapid and occurs in people with an extreme sensitivity to a particular substance, e.g. nuts or penicillin.

Keywords: Collapse/pathology

Angina pectoris

Angina is Latin for tight chest. This condition results in chest pain due to insufficient oxygen being carried in the heart muscle in the blood. Can be brought on by physical exertion or stress. The most common cause of angina is the thickening of the arteries caused by fatty deposits.

Keyword: Collapse

Angle's classification of occlusion

An orthodontic examination assesses the jaw relationship and determines which class of occlusion an individual has and if orthodontic treatment is required to correct the bite. The classifications are categorised as:

Class I: normal jaw relationship.

Class II, division I: protruding upper incisors, overjet is increased.

Class II, division II: upper central incisors are tilted backwards, overjet decreased, overbite increased.

Class III: prominent chin, overjet absent or reverse.

Keyword: Orthodontics

Ankylosis

The root of a deciduous tooth has become cemented to the alveolar bone resulting in failed exfoliation of the tooth resulting in natural loss. A surgical extraction is required to remove the root.

Keyword: Surgical extractions

Anodontia

This is the absence of six or more teeth. The teeth buds may be absent at birth or damaged whilst developing due to infection or disease.

Keyword: Anatomy

Anterior superior dental nerve

A branch of the maxillary division providing nerve supply to incisors, canines and the labial gingiva.

Keyword: Anatomy

A

Anterior open bite

This is determined after an orthodontic examination to record the size and position of the teeth and jaw. In this case, the incisors do not meet when biting.

Keyword: Orthodontics

Antibiotic cover

This is given to people one hour prior to treatment if they have congenital heart defects, artificial heart valves or a history of rheumatic fever. This precautionary measure is to prevent infective endocarditis.

Keyword: Drugs

Antibiotics

Drugs used to treat infections caused by bacteria. They are administered internally to kill bacteria and prevent bacterial infection in cases of immune system impairment.

Keyword: Drugs

Antibodies

These are contained in plasma and give resistance to disease. An antibody is released by certain white blood cells and can overcome bacteria. Antibodies may be formed in response to vaccines providing immunity.

Keyword: Pathology

Anticoagulants

Drugs which are used for people who are at risk of blood clots. They may bleed excessively after treatment as a result of taking these drugs as they suppress the capacity of the blood to clot.

Keyword: Drugs

Antitoxins

Just like antibodies these are contained in plasma and work together in fighting bacteria. Antitoxins neutralise any bacteria and if infection returns, it is immediately overcome by the antitoxins already present.

Keyword: Pathology

A

Antrum

Known also as a maxillary sinus, it is situated on either side of the nasal cavity where the maxilla is hollow. Complications may arise during an extraction resulting in a root being pushed inside the antrum so it is of great importance to know its location.

Keyword: Anatomy

Anus

This is the end of the alimentary tract where faeces are expelled from the body which is open only during defecation. It is situated at the end of the alimentary canal.

Keyword: Anatomy

Aorta

The body's main artery, supplying oxygenated blood to all other parts. It is large in diameter and has a thick wall enabling it to cope with high pressure and volume of blood.

Keyword: Anatomy

Apex locator

This is an electronic device that is used in endodontic (root canal treatment) procedures. It determines the distance to the apical foramen. A file is attached to the tip and when it is within 1 mm of the apex, the device will beep.

Keyword: Endodontic

Apicectomy

This is done as a last resort in order to save a tooth that has had a failed root filling or if it was not possible to do one. It is an operation to remove an infected apex and surrounding tissues. If this procedure fails, the next step is to extract the tooth.

Keyword: Minor oral surgery

Applicators

Can be metal which can be sterilised in the autoclave, or disposable. They are used for applying material such as bonding agents or linings intra-orally.

Keyword: Restorations/instruments

Aprons

A

Disposable aprons can be worn when cleaning instruments to protect the worker's uniform from splatter. Aprons can also be worn during clinical procedures such as extractions and disposed after use with every patient to prevent cross-infection. There are various types available and in hospitals or when maintaining a surgical environment in the dental surgery, disposable gowns can be worn.

Keyword: Cross-infection control

Archwire

Used in orthodontic procedures whilst fitting a fixed appliance. Brackets are cemented to each tooth and the archwire is secured onto each one. This provides the force required to position the teeth over a period of time.

Keyword: Orthodontics

Artery

A blood vessel that carries blood away from the heart. The largest artery is the aorta, which is systemic and carries blood, pumped from the left ventricle to all parts of the body. Pulmonary arteries carry blood from the right ventricle to the lungs.

Keyword: Anatomy

Articaine

A local anaesthetic given internally by injection, usually supplied as 4% articaine, 1:200,000 epinephrine. This solution is administered to prolong anaesthesia during lengthy procedures.

Keyword: Drugs

Articular eminence

The ridge part of the glenoid fossa which is situated in the temporal bone.

Keyword: Anatomy

Articulator

This piece of equipment mimics jaw movements when underlying models and wax rims are mounted onto it. The work is sent to a laboratory to construct a denture for the wax try-in stage of the process.

Keyword: Prosthetics

Articulating paper
This is held in place by Miller forceps to check occlusion. The patient bites onto the paper and a mark will be left on the tooth surface if there is a high spot to indicate that adjustments need to be made to correct the bite.

Keywords: Prosthetics/restoration

Asepsis
Agents that are used to eliminate bacteria, fungi, viruses and spores maintain an operative field in surgery preventing cross-infection. This procedure reduces the risk of bacterial contamination.

Keyword: Cross-infection control

Aspirator
Also known as suction. Chairside assistance is given by the nurse holding a tube which is inserted into an attachment in the suction unit. This is then used to suction saliva, blood or any other debris from the patient's mouth. It also acts as a retractor, protecting soft tissues and providing a clear field of view for the operator.

Keyword: Moisture control

Aspirin
An analgesic used to relieve minor aches and pains. Can reduce fever, is an anti-inflammatory and has a blood thinning effect.

Keyword: Drugs

Asthma
A common disease that causes the airways of the lungs to tighten, causing symptoms such as wheezing, coughing, difficulty in breathing and chest pain. Attacks can be triggered by dust, smoke, chemicals and pollution. Medication is available to relieve symptoms.

Keyword: Pathology

Atrium
Situated in the upper compartments of the heart, left and right. The right atrium receives blood returning from all parts of the

body except the lungs. The left atrium receives oxygenated blood from the lungs in the pulmonary vein.

Keywords: Heart and circulation

Attrition
A cause of tooth surface loss. Occlusal surfaces are gradually worn away or flattened by friction or abrasion; the most common cause is grinding or bruxism.

Keyword: Dental disease

Autoclave
Used for the sterilisation of instruments. Vacuum autoclaves require instruments to be packaged and non-vacuum allows instruments to be kept on an open tray. The sterilisation cycles ensure that all pathogenic organisms and spores are killed by the autoclave heating up to 134°C.

Keywords: Cross-infection control/sterilisation

Autoclave tape
This can be written on to indicate which instruments belong to whom and can be placed on the tray of instruments or sterilisation pouch to indicate the contents. The tape will change colour to show evidence of a successful cycle.

Keyword: Sterilisation

Automatic film processor
Also known as x-ray developer. An x-ray is unwrapped and the film is fed into the machine whilst being protected from light. The film is transported on rollers and conveyors and passed through solutions of developer, fixer, water and is then dried to produce an image.

Keyword: Radiography

Austin retractor
An instrument used in surgical procedures and acts as a retractor and protector of soft tissues. It enables a clear field of vision for the operator.

Keyword: Surgical instruments

Avulsed tooth

This is when a tooth is knocked out due to trauma. If the periodontal ligament is vital, the tooth can be pushed back into the socket. After the tooth has become dislodged it needs to be kept moist and immediately placed in the socket in order for this to be successful.

Keyword: Minor oral surgery

Azithromycin

An antibiotic derived from erythromycin. Used only for antibiotic cover for people who are penicillin allergic.

Keyword: Drugs

B

Bacillus fusiformis
A bacteria found in acute necrotising ulcerative gingivitis.

Keyword: Pathology

Bacteraemia
This is the presence of bacteria circulating in the blood and can occur most commonly during extractions and scaling.

Keyword: Pathology

Bacteria
Microscopic single-celled organisms which are subdivided into groups according to their shape. Some bacteria are beneficial and harmless and others can cause disease.

Keyword: Pathology

Band removers
Orthodontic instrument used for removing molar bands from each tooth.

Keyword: Orthodontics

Barrier (non-permeable)
Comes in various shapes and sizes to cover instruments, chairs, handles, hoses, light switches and handpieces. They are used to prevent cross-contamination by permitting passage of liquid and are changed after every patient and disposed of.

Keyword: Cross-infection control

Basic life support (BLS)
To supply oxygenated blood to an unconscious person's brain and heart by means of artificial respiration. This can keep a person alive whilst waiting for medical assistance.

Keyword: Collapse

Bayonet
A type of extraction forceps used for removing upper wisdom teeth and roots. They are easily recognised by their elongated beak making it easier to access the upper 8s.

Keyword: Minor oral surgery

Beebee crown shears
Scissors-like instrument with short blades used for trimming temporary crowns.

Keyword: Restorations

Bile
This is secreted by the liver and carries away waste products. It is a greenish-brown liquid stored in the gall bladder and also helps to break down fats in the small intestine for digestion.

Keyword: Digestion

Biopsy
The surgical removal of tissue or cells sent to a pathology lab for diagnostic testing of possible disease. An excisional biopsy is to remove the whole abnormal area and incisional is to remove a small sample.

Keyword: Minor oral surgery

Biopsy specimen
After a soft tissue investigation, the biopsy tissue is sent for further investigation to a pathology lab for diagnostic opinion. The specimen container is usually provided by the laboratory on request. It contains a special solution so it needs to be water tight and leak-proof. The container needs to be wrapped in absorbent material in case of breakage. The container will have a label ensuring that all the necessary details are included. The specimen container is then placed in a padded envelope and posted to the lab.

Keyword: Minor oral surgery/pathology

Bisecting angle technique
An x-ray film is placed intra-orally. This technique is used if there are restrictions such as size of patient's mouth or poor access.

Bisected means that the angle at which the x-ray is taken is halved to provide a true image of the tooth's length and width.

Keyword: Radiography

B

Bite registration paste
Different types and thickness are available to determine a person's occlusal relationship.

Keyword: Prosthetics/restorations

Bitewing radiograph
Intra-oral x-ray which provides an image of premolars and molars on the right or left side of the mouth. Usually taken on the first visit and the repeated every two to three years depending on the individual's decay rate.

Keyword: Radiography

BiTine ring
These can be sterilised in the autoclave and hold a disposable sectional matrix in place around the tooth. The BiTine ring is held in a tweezers-like instrument holder and positioned around the tooth.

Keyword: Restorations

Black's classification
This is the classification of cavities and fillings. There are five classes depending on the surface.

Keyword: Restorations

Blake's knife
Surgical instrument used to remove gingival tissue during a gingivectomy procedure. The blade is disposable and can vary in size and shape.

Keyword: Minor oral surgery

Blank film
An x-ray once developed can appear blank. This can be caused by failing to switch on x-ray equipment meaning that the film has not been exposed and a blank film has been processed. If mistakes are made during manual processing by placing the film in fixer first, this also produces a blank film.

Keyword: Radiography

Bleaching
This is done to lighten discoloured teeth and the procedure can be done using several methods either in a surgery or at home.

Keyword: Cosmetic dentistry

Blood
Adults have about five litres of blood which is pumped by the heart and circulates through veins, arteries and capillaries at a constant temperature of 37°C.

Keyword: Heart and circulation

Blood pressure
This can vary between individuals. When the heart contracts, a reading (systolic, top number) is measured of the blood pressure in the arteries. The diastolic (bottom number) is the resting measurements. An average, healthy adult's blood pressure should be about 120/80.

Keyword: Physiology

Blood spillage
If blood is spilled from a container or as a result from an operation procedure, it needs to be dealt with immediately. The blood should be covered with paper towels and treated with 10,000 ppm sodium hypochlorite solution or sodium dichloroisocyanurate granules. After five minutes the towels can be cleared and disposed in clinical waste. PPE must be worn when dealing with this and ventilation is required.

Keyword: Cross-infection control

Blue ring conventional handpiece
A slow speed handpiece attached to a motor running at a speed of 40,000 rpm. Latch grip burs and prophy cups are attached to it.

Keyword: Handpiece and burs

Blunt scissors
These get confused with surgical scissors. They are used for cutting, as one side is pointed. The blunt side prevents trauma to any soft tissues.

Keyword: Instruments

Blurred film
An x-ray can appear as blurred if movement of the film has occurred during exposure for example if the patient moved his or her head.

Keyword: Radiography

Boley gauge
A measuring device used mainly in laboratories but sometimes used in clinics as well. The device measures the thickness of dental materials.

Keyword: Prosthetics

Bonding agents
Available in a range of products allowing filling materials to bond/adhere to dentine and enamel.

Keyword: Restorations

Bone
The material that the skeleton is made of. This provides the framework that protects internal organs. Bone has several layers containing blood vessels, nerves and cells.

Keywords: Anatomy and physiology

Bone file
A surgical chisel-like instrument used to file and smooth away any alveolar bone which remains after an extraction.

Keyword: Minor oral surgery

Bone nibblers
A surgical instrument with a spring mechanism between the handles. Its sharpened working end is used to trim sharp edges of bone.

Keyword: Minor oral surgery

Bone replacement material
This material is exogenous, derived from another source, it is bovine/cow derived and is used as a bone replacement to create new bone whilst placing a dental implant (bone grafting) if natural bone is insufficient to support the implant. Bone can also

be used from the patient's own bone, known as autogenous bone or bone from another human known as allogenous bone.

Keyword: Implants

Bone resorption

This is the loss of substance from teeth such as dentine, alveolar bone, cementum. Primary teeth are lost by this process. Resorption of the roots means that the teeth become loose. After an extraction, osteoclast cells eat away at the alveolar bone reducing the alveolar ridge.

Keyword: Anatomy

Bone rongeurs

A surgical stainless steel instrument used for the trimming of sharp edges of bone which can remain after an extraction. This is achieved by using the sharpened working end; they can be used anywhere in the mouth.

Keyword: Minor oral surgery

Bone trap

This special suction device is used during surgical procedures to collect patient's natural bone whilst drilling. It is collected in a special filter part of the aspirator and can be used as a bone substitute if the patient is having an implant placed and their own bone in the placement area is of poor quality. This natural bone can then be placed to provide support for the implant.

Keyword: Implants

Borrelia vincenti

A spiral, elongated bacteria which is another contributor to acute necrotising ulcerative gingivitis.

Keyword: Microbiology

Bottle brush

Can be autoclaved after it has been used to clean inside non-disposable suction tubes that have not had a successful ultrasonic clean.

Keyword: Cross-infection control

Bowdler-Henry rake retractor

This surgical instrument retracts the gum flap during a surgical procedure. It enables the operator to have a clear field of vision and protects the soft tissues.

Keyword: Minor oral surgery

Bracket holders

Used in orthodontic treatment, they hold the ortho bracket securely in place whilst positioning it onto the tooth for cement fixture.

Keyword: Orthodontics

Bracket removers

An orthodontic instrument that is used to take the brackets off teeth. They are stainless steel and have a tweezers-like function. The instrument inserts into the bracket enabling it to be lifted off carefully. There is also a plastic version of the instrument which is shaped like a gun and has replacement wires which lift off the brackets.

Keyword: Orthodontics

Briault probe

Used during a dental examination. Using its angled working ends it is used to detect caries on mesial and distal surfaces.

Keyword: Examination/oral health

Bridge

A prosthetic laboratory-made appliance used as a fixed replacement for a missing tooth or several teeth, bridging the gap. The replacement tooth is called a pontic and the supporting tooth is called an abutment. The crowns on the abutments are called retainers. There are different types of bridges depending on the requirements of the patient. In some cases the bridge can have a joint incorporated in the design, this is called a dovetail joint and allows some degree of flexibility. A bridge is a natural choice to fill in the space in a mouth due to missing teeth. If the space is left unfilled then the surrounding teeth could drift out of position causing problems with the bite, gums and decay.

Keyword: Prosthetics

Broach
An endodontic disposable instrument used for removing the pulp by the barbs of wire snagging it. They come in different sizes and widths.

Keyword: Endodontic

B

Bronchi
These branch off from the trachea and divide into the right and left bronchus to enter the right and left lungs.

Keyword: Respiration

Brook airway
A tube which fits into a person's mouth providing expired air ventilation. The tube is blown into by the operator. A valve prevents expired air from reaching the operator which may contain blood or vomit from the victim.

Keyword: Collapse

Bruxism
Also known as tooth grinding or clenching. Most commonly done during sleep, therefore the person may be unaware of this. It is recognised by excessive wear on the teeth. Can be triggered by stress.

Keyword: Anatomy

Buccal canine retractor
Used during orthodontic treatment, this spring is placed buccally around the canine to enable distal and palatal movement to correct malocclusion.

Keyword: Orthodontics

Buccal sulcus
Buccal is Latin for cheek. This is simply the space between the teeth and the mucous membrane lining of the cheeks.

Keyword: Anatomy

Buccal tooth surface
This is the tooth surface of the molars and pre-molars facing the cheeks.

Keyword: Anatomy

B

Buccinator

This is the muscle of the cheek attached above and below to the buccal surface of the alveolar process of each jaw. It also works with the muscles of mastication.

Keyword: Anatomy

Buffer action

This is the antacid function of saliva neutralising acid from sugary food or drink.

Keyword: Caries

Burning mouth syndrome

This describes pain or discomfort in the mouth affecting the tongue, lips, cheeks and other parts of the skin inside of the mouth. Patients complain of a burning or scalding feeling. The condition mainly affects women after menopause but men can get it too. Thrush infections, blood or vitamin deficiencies can be the cause as can hormonal changes, stress, anxiety or depression. Thorough examinations and blood tests will be done to eliminate cancer as the cause. Once reassurance is given of no serious disorders then symptoms usually ease.

Keyword: Pathology

Burnisher

Comes in various sizes of working ends. Used as a filling instrument it smooths the filling material once in place and condenses the amalgam in the prepared cavity.

Keyword: Restorations

Burs

Come in various shapes and sizes and attach to the air rotor handpice, slow speed handpiece or any other handpiece unit. The many functions include: cutting, polishing, finishing and trimming teeth, fillings, prosthetics, and metal. Can be used in endodontics. They can be disposable or sterilised in an autoclave.

Keyword: Handpieces and burs

Bur block

Used to store burs. There are different types available and are used to keep burs organised. Some can be sterilised in an autoclave.

Keyword: Burs

Bur brush

Many types and sizes available used to clean debris off burrs when ultrasonic cleaning has not been affective. They can be sterilised in an autoclave.

Keyword: Cross-infection control

C

Calcium
A mineral that is essential for cell function, muscle contraction, blood clotting and maintaining healthy bones and teeth. Calcium is present in dairy products, eggs and leafy green vegetables.

Keyword: Digestion

Calcium hydroxide
Comes in a powder and liquid which requires some mixing, or in a paste. It is used to line a cavity before a filling is placed. It is non-irritating and can be used in endodontic procedures as well.

Keyword: Restoration

Calculus
Also called tartar, this is the hard residue that can form on teeth if oral hygiene is poor. It starts as soft plaque which produces mineral salts and, when mixed with saliva, hardens over time if not removed. It is yellowish in colour and will need removing by a dental care professional to stop the periodontal disease process.

Keyword: Periodontal Disease

Candida albicans
This fungus is the most common one found in the mouth. This organism is associated with other oral conditions such as thrush. Antifungal drugs can be prescribed to treat these infections.

Keyword: Microbiology

Canine
Two in the upper jaw and two in the lower jaw. These are single cusped teeth, pointed and usually have one root. They are located between the incisors and premolars.

Keyword: Anatomy

Cannula
A tube that is inserted into a blood vessel, lymphatic vessel or body cavity. They are used to withdraw or introduce fluids. During a dental procedure it is used during intravenous sedation to introduce the tranquilliser. The cannula is inserted into a vein on the top of the hand.

Keyword: Conscious sedation

Cantilever bridge
This is a fixed prosthetic appliance placed if there are teeth only on one side of the span. The retaining teeth are usually those immediately to one side of the pontic. The retaining natural teeth act as anchors for the pontic which replaces the missing teeth, bridging the gap.

Keyword: Prosthetics

Capillary
This is a thin walled vessel through which blood passes. This enables the blood and cells to exchange oxygen, glucose, carbon dioxide and water.

Keyword: Heart and circulation

Carbohydrate
This provides the body with a source of fuel (energy). Foods such as sugar, flour, vegetables and oats contain carbohydrates.

Keyword: Digestion

Cardiac arrest
A sudden halt and loss of heart function. The most common cause is heart attack. The symptoms are collapse, loss of consciousness, absent pulse, and laboured breathing. Immediate action must be taken to make the heart beat artificially.

Keyword: Collapse

Cardiopulmonary resuscitation (CPR)
If a person has had a cardiac arrest, then life saving measures need to be administered whilst waiting for the emergency services. Mouth to mouth is given, if this fails, chest compressions are done to restore blood circulation to the brain.

Keyword: Health and safety/emergency procedures

C

Caries
This is tooth decay caused mainly by plaque from food deposits. The decay will gradually erode the enamel and dentine. If not detected early it can invade the pulp.

Keyword: Oral disease

Cartilage
This is an elastic, tough type of connective tissue performing several functions. It covers the surface of joints allowing bones to slide over one another preventing friction and acts as a shock absorber.

Keyword: Anatomy

Carver
Double- or single-ended filling instrument. They are often referred to by their proper names of Cleoid carver, Hollenbach carver and Wards carver. Available in various shapes and sizes and used to shape a filling and carve any excess material to reduce the height of the newly placed filing.

Keyword: Basic instrument

Castroviejo needle holders
Used during minor oral surgery to hold the suture needle securely. They look like scissors and have serrated edges for grip.

Keyword: Minor oral surgery

Cellulitis
This is an infection of the skin most commonly caused by Streptococci bacteria and can affect an infected tooth; treated with antibiotics.

Keyword: Anatomy

Celluloid matrix
Used when doing composite fillings to ensure a good contact point. They are supplied as transparent strips and are single use.

Keyword: Restoration

Cementum
This is a calcified substance, very similar to bone, that surrounds the root of a tooth, providing a protective outer covering.

Keyword: Anatomy

Cephalometric radiograph
An extra-oral radiograph providing the image of the skull, side and frontal views, used mainly in orthodontic assessments to allow measurements to be taken.

Keyword: Radiography

Cephalostat
This is an extra-oral view used in radiography, similar to an orthopantomograph (OPG) machine giving a full view of both jaws. This is used in specialist orthodontics.

Keyword: Radiography

Charting
Prescribed in the form of a diagram representing all of the teeth. The chart is numbered and divided into upper and lower arches, left and right. A patient's chart is used to show missing and present teeth and any other work that has been done or needs to be done.

Keyword: Anatomy

Cheek retractors
Come in various shapes and sizes used to retract cheeks during procedures such as fixing veneers, bonding appliances and taking photos of teeth to allow good visibility.

Keyword: Instruments

Chisel
This instrument is used during extraction and surgical procedures to elevate and loosen a tooth from the periodontal ligament. There are different sizes available.

Keyword: Instruments

Chlorhexidine
Available as an antiseptic mouthwash or as disinfectant solution. Should only be used for a short period of time under the instruction of a dental care professional as it stains teeth. It helps to keep the mouth clean and prevent plaque formation.

Keyword: Drugs

Chrome cobalt
The base of this denture is made from metal rather than acrylic. This makes it thinner to help prevent the patient from gagging. It may also last longer.

Keyword: Prosthetics

Chronic periodontitis
This is a result of untreated gingivitis. Bacteria attack the periodontal tissues which surround the tooth which may cause tooth loss.

Keyword: Periodontal dsease

Circulatory system
This is the maintenance of continuous blood flow throughout the body provided by the heart and blood vessels. This is divided into further parts, see Coronary, Pulmonary artery and vein, and Systemic.

Keyword: Heart and circulation

Citanest
See Prilocaine.

Cleft palate
This birth defect is a result of abnormal facial development causing a split to occur in the palate, which can occur together with a split in the upper lip. The vertical split in the upper lip is usually off-centre. The upper gum may also be cleft and the nose will appear crooked. The gap in the cleft palate can extend from the back of the palate to the teeth. Surgery to correct this is usually done soon after birth and further surgery, such as orthodontics and speech therapy, may be required later on.

Keyword: Orthodontics

Clindamycin

This is an antibiotic used if patients are allergic to penicillin type drugs. It is given by injection or taken orally and is used for the prevention of infective carditis.

Keyword: Drugs

Clinical audit

An audit can be carried out on different aspects of the practice, for example infection control. This will ensure that high standards of practice are met and maintained. This is a quality assurance system that is required in all NHS practices, an essential feature of clinical governance.

Keyword: Health and safety

Clinical waste

This includes all waste produced at the practice that has been contaminated with blood, saliva or any other body fluid. The waste is categorised and disposed of in a correct manner. There are regulations to follow to ensure safety. The waste should be stored correctly and collected by a certified company.

Keyword: Health and safety/Cross-infection control

Compomer

This material acts as a composite and glass ionomer cement combined. It comes premixed and ready to be placed in the prepared cavity and provides a fluoride release. The material chemically bonds to the tooth surface.

Keyword: Filling

Composite

A tooth-coloured restoration, comes in various types and shades to be placed in anterior and posterior teeth. The tooth surface is etched and bonded and the composite placed and set by a curing light.

Keyword: Restoration

Condyle

This is situated in the mandible and is the rounded bone used for articulation with another bone. You can feel the bone when you open and close your mouth. The Latin word condyle translates into knuckle.

Keyword: Anatomy

Conical drill

This is a flared (cone shaped) drill used as a final drill in the preparation of an osteotomy site of implant placement. Not all implant manufactures have this and the use depends on the shape of the implant. Astra is one system where it is used.

Keyword: Implant

Coning

This fault can occur during radiography during exposure. This means that the operator has not centralised the tube head of the x-ray machine onto the film causing partial loss of image.

Keyword: Radiography

Conscious sedation

This technique will provide a relaxed state for the patient by the use of sedative drugs. The patient will remain conscious which will enable the operator to carry out the procedure starting with the administration of local anaesthetic.

Keyword: Sedation

Consent

This can be verbal or written and a record must be kept, notes written and a signature obtained. An exam or any other treatment carried out requires informed consent from the patient.

Keyword: Records/administration

Contact point

This is the point between adjoining teeth where the tooth contacts the next tooth.

Keyword: Anatomy

Contaminated

This term refers to anything that has come into contact with blood, saliva or any other body fluid. This could mean a risk of cross-infection unless standard precautions were applied.

Keyword: Cross-infection control

Continuing professional development (CPD)

This is a compulsory system of life long learning which all professionals complementary to dentistry (PCD) are required to do to develop new skills and update knowledge. The GDC has proposed how many hours of CPD are required.

Keyword: Development of knowledge

Controlled area

This area surrounding the x-ray equipment is normally within 1.5 metres of an x-ray beam. When x-rays are taken, individuals should be prevented from entering this controlled area. Staff are advised to stand 1.5–2 metres from the x-ray tube out of the direction of the primary beam.

Keyword: Radiology

Controlled waste regulations

This regulation is governed by the Environmental Protection Act to ensure that all waste used in the dental practice is disposed of correctly and collected by a registered company. Waste is categorised and should be separated accordingly, for example sharps, amalgam and special waste.

Keyword: Waste disposal/health and safety

Control of Substances Hazardous to Health Regulations (COSHH)

Any hazardous substances used on the premises needs to be identified and an assessment made. Records should be kept of procedures and precautions to follow to reduce the risk as much as possible. This is a regulation which comes under the Health and safety at work Act.

Keyword: Health and safety

Conventional handpiece

Used as a slow or low speed handpiece, they are contra-angled enabling access to every tooth, and are used with latch grip attachments. The functions include removing caries and polishing. A smaller head called a miniature can be attached to the handpiece when treating smaller mouths.

Keyword: Handpieces and burs

Collagen membrane
This tissue is derived from pigs and can be used in conjunction with a bone replacement material whilst placing a dental implant. This will enable the new bone to slowly grow into the patient's natural bone.

Keyword: Implants

College tweezers
Used to pick up objects and place objects in the mouth. They can lock to help prevent dropping the object.

Keyword: Instruments

Coloured identification rings
These come in various types, sizes and colours and are placed on instruments for organisation, coding and identification.

Keyword: Instruments

Composite gun
The composite capsule is inserted into the gun and used by the operator to deliver the material onto the tooth surface.

Keyword: Fillings

Composite polishing strip
Used interproximally to polish and smooth any rough bits of cured composite material. Can also be used to clean interdental stain.

Keyword: Fillings

Contact former
Comes in various shapes and sizes. Used during a composite filling procedure to allow good interproximal contact between adjacent teeth. The instrument is placed on the composite during the curing stage.

Keyword: Filling instrument

Coons ligature pliers
Used in orthodontic procedures to tie ligatures into a figure of eight. The angle size of the beak varies with each instrument.

Keyword: Orthodontic

Cord packer
Looks like a large excavator and is serrated. Used simply to pack cord of varying sizes into the gingival margin before taking an impression for a prosthetic to be made. This ensures the prosthetic will fit right up to the gum.

Keyword: Instruments

Coronary artery
Either of two main arteries supplying the tissue of the heart with oxygenated blood, commonly referred to as the left or right main coronary arteries.

Keyword: Pathology

Coronary thrombosis
Also known as a blood clot when one of the coronary arteries has a blockage, resulting in a section of the heart being deprived of oxygen.

Keyword: Pathology

Coronoid process
This is the sharp triangular projection of bone situated on the top of the ramus.

Keyword: Anatomy

Corrosive substance
If a corrosive substance is used incorrectly it may cause damage to the skin, tissues, eyes and any other parts of the body on contact. Inhalation of a corrosive substance can damage the respiratory tract. Acids are the most common corrosive substances used.

Keyword: Health and safety

Corticosteroid
Mainly prescribed in dentistry as an antiinflammatory drug as pain relief and to promote the healing of mouth ulcers. Applied externally.

Keyword: Drugs

Cotton pellets
Used to control moisture. Held in place by tweezers to absorb blood, saliva or dental materials. Can be used to smooth a restoration and a temporary dressing.

Keyword: Restorations

Cotton rolls
Used for moisture control and to retract any soft tissues to give a clear field of vision.

Keyword: Restorations

Cover screw
Used during a dental implant placement to cover the implant whilst healing takes place. They are made of titanium and come in various heights.

Keyword: Implants

Cowhorn extraction forceps
Used for extracting left and right lower molars. The beak is pointed and designed to grip the molar.

Keyword: Extraction instrument

Cranium
This is one of the three regions of the skull surrounding the brain. It is made up of six plates of bone which interlock with each other.

Keyword: Anatomy

Cresophene
An antiseptic endodontic medicament placed on a cotton pellet or paper point which is then used in a temporary dressing to kill bacteria before a root filling is carried out.

Keyword: Endodontic

Creutzfeldt-Jakob disease (CJD)
This illness affects the nervous system causing damage to the brain. It is caused by a prion protein that contaminates the nervous system. The prion protein is very similar to a virus by the way it replicates itself, causing the disease, however, this protein is tougher than a virus. It cannot be destroyed

and at present there is no cure. There are four types of CJD: sporadic CJD, iatrogenic CJD, familial or genetic CJD and variant CJD.

Keyword: Pathology

Cricothyrotomy

An emergency procedure performed to relieve the blockage/obstruction in the airway if all other measures fail. The cannula needed to do this is found in the emergency drug kit. Oxygen supply is connected to the needle which is inserted into the larynx.

Keyword: Emergency procedure

Crohn's disease

An inflammatory bowel disease causing abdominal pain, anaemia, diarrhoea and weight loss. The condition can cause complications in other parts of the body, such as arthritis in the joints.

Keyword: Medical condition

Cross bite

This discrepancy is determined by an orthodontic exam. The upper posterior teeth bite inside the lower teeth rather than outside them. This can be corrected over time with the use of a special orthodontic appliance.

Keyword: Orthodontic

Cross infection

This is the transmission of infection from various sources, for example blood or saliva from one person to another, e.g. from patient to staff or staff to patient. This can happen if standard precautions are not applied.

Keyword: Health and safety/cross-infection control

Crown

There are various types of these laboratory made artificial restorations. They can be a permanent or temporary fixture. The tooth is prepared during a crown preparation procedure ready to receive the fixture once made at the lab. The crown will fit over the remainder of the tooth using cement. Crowns are usually

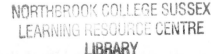

fitted to a tooth that is heavily restored, root filled or for aesthetic reasons.

Keyword: Restoration

Crown forms
Various types available depending on which tooth is going to be covered. They are used as a temporary measure, fixed by temporary cement whilst the permanent crown is being made.

Keyword: Prosthetics

Crown remover
Used to remove cemented crowns by placing the beak of the instrument at the gingival margin of the crown whilst gently tapping the weighted handle a few times to loosen the fixture.

Keyword: Prosthetics instrument

Cryers
Used in minor oral surgery to remove bone and loosen root tips. They have one working end, left or right orientated and are of different sizes.

Keyword: Minor oral surgery

Curette
Used in periodontal procedures and varies in size and shape depending on which area of the mouth the instrument is being used. They are used to remove calculus, plaque and stain. Used for deep scaling procedures.

Keyword: Periodontal

Curing light
This piece of equipment is used to harden material using halogen or LED. The light will cure composite, bonds and sealants. A protective shield should be used to shade eyes from the light.

Keyword: Restorations

Cusp of Carabelli
This is the name of the extra cusp that upper first molars often have on their mesio-palatal surface.

Keyword: Anatomy

Custom tray

Also know as a special tray. Primary impressions using standard trays are taken of the patient's mouth and sent to the laboratory where this tray is made from an acrylic material to fit the individual's mouth. This will provide a final accurate impression for dentures to be made.

Keyword: Prosthetics

C

Cyanosis

This can occur if there is too much deoxygenated haemoglobin in the blood or if a patient has a heart or lung disorder. When monitoring patients during treatment and you notice a change in colour from pink to purple on their face, lips, fingers or ears, you need to alert the operator immediately. The patient may also appear pale and be sweating.

Keyword: Health and safety

Cyst

An abnormal swelling or lump, most of the time harmless. This sac of fluid can vary depending on which part of the body it is situated. When in the jaw and left untreated it can enlarge causing problems.

Keyword: Minor oral surgery

D

Data Protection Act (1998)

This act provides regulations relating to the processing of information. Personal data of patients and staff must be protected and secured in the workplace. All information is to remain confidential to protect the individual from persons not authorised to access details. Only data that are required should only be collected and not discussed with other parties without consent. Individuals have the right to access their own information. Personal information must not be stored for any longer than necessary or required by law.

Keyword: Confidentiality

Deciduous teeth

Also known as primary teeth, temporary teeth, milk or baby teeth. These are the first set of teeth that usually start to erupt at the age of six months onwards. There are twenty of them, ten in the upper and ten in the lower jaw and will start to be replaced by permanent teeth from about the age of six.

Keyword: Anatomy

Decontamination

This is the cleaning and sterilisation of instruments and equipment contaminated with oral fluids, other body fluids (blood or saliva), hazardous substances or infectious organisms that can cause infection. The decontamination process prevents cross-infection and all practices should apply standard precautions.

Keyword: Cross-infection control

Defibrillator
Medical equipment used only by a trained person during a cardiac emergency. The electric shocks are the most effective way to return normal rhythm to a heart.

Keyword: Collapse

Demineralisation
This occurs due to acidic conditions in the mouth. If the pH level in the mouth drops from its normal level of pH7, then the acids produced from the bacteria will form an abnormal loss of mineral salts in the saliva, preventing it from neutralising the acids. Eventually this will cause mineral loss in the enamel.

Keyword: Oral disease

Dental fibrils
These are discovered under a microscope and are present in odontoblasts which form the dentine. They pass into the dentine through tubules working as a link with the pulp to respond to irritation or any damage to the dentine.

Keyword: Anatomy

Dental health education
Making individuals aware of the causes and prevention of dental disease. Advising the individual on how to maintain a healthy mouth by having regular check-ups with a GDP or hygienist as well as toothbrush instruction and diet advice.

Keyword: Prevention of disease

Dental Practice Board (DPB)
Now called the Dental Services Provision under the NHS Business Services Authority (BSA). Responsible for providing the GDP with payment of treatment fees. This can be done online when the data is collated to ensure timely payments. They will also answer any queries regarding Data Protection Act and Freedom of Information Act.

Keyword: Administration

Dentine
This is the layer of the tooth that lies beneath the enamel; its hard tissue surrounds the pulp. The enamel protects the dentine from

stimuli. Dentine is a living tissue, slightly elastic and yellowish in colour.

Keyword: Anatomy

Dentine pins
Used for added retention in large cavities before filling material is placed. The pins are drilled into the remaining crown structure. Bonding agents can be used for retention also.

Keyword: Restoration

Dentino-enamel junction
See Amelo-dentinal junction

Keyword: Anatomy

Dentists Act
This act ensures high standards of professional conduct amongst all professionals complementary to dentistry (PCD). Anyone who is registered with the General Dental Council (GDC) and found guilty of a criminal offence or serious professional misconduct can be removed from the register.

Keyword: Governing body

Dentures
Removable, artificial prosthesis replacing missing teeth. Can be a full set of dentures or partial and made in different materials. Worn by an individual to restore normal appearances and to enable mastication and clear speech.

Keyword: Dentures/prosthetic

Denture stomatitis
Also known as denture sore mouth. It is a common oral condition associated with a fungal infection. The condition will appear on the soft tissue that the denture covers, becoming swollen and red. This may be caused by dentures not being cleaned properly.

Keyword: Microbiology

Dermatitis
If present this presents as a red, scaly, itchy rash on the skin. This can occur from an allergy to a substance which has been in direct

contact with the skin. Dermatitis can also be caused by stress. It can be treated with corticosteroid drugs.

Keyword: Pathology

Developer
A hazardous solution used in the first stage of processing an x-ray film. This produces the image on the film and then it has to go through further timed stages until complete for viewing. The developer is changed very carefully at regular intervals whilst protective clothing is worn.

Keyword: Radiography

D

Diabetes
There are different types of this disease and it occurs when the body cannot make or use insulin correctly. The insulin hormone turns sugar in food we eat into energy. If a person has this illness, then too much sugar can stay in the blood damaging different parts of the body. Diabetes can be controlled through diet or medication. Whilst treating diabetic patients, it is important to know if they have had their insulin (if required) or if they have eaten. They will need monitoring throughout the treatment.

Keyword: Disease

Diagnostic radiograph
Taken during endodontic treatment to determine the length of the root enabling the preparation of the canal. The correct length of instrument needs to be used to avoid apical perforation.

Keyword: Endodontic

Diamond bur
Various shapes and sizes used in the air/high speed turbine for cutting the enamel surface, dentine and removing old filling material.

Keyword: Handpieces and burs

Diaphragm
Plays an important role in breathing. This dome shaped sheet of muscle separates the chest from the abdomen. Air is drawn into

the lungs by the muscle fibres contracting and pulling the diaphragm downwards.

Keyword: Anatomy

Diastema
This simply means the gap between the upper central incisors.

Keyword: Anatomy

Diazepam
A drug which is used short term to treat anxiety and insomnia
and relax muscles. Some nervous patients are prescribed this
drug by their doctor or dentist to alleviate anxiety before treatment. It does have side effects and should be used with
caution.

Keyword: Drugs

Digestion
This is a process involved in the breaking down of food so it can
be transported and used by the body.

Keyword: Digestion

Digestive system
This contains a group of organs responsible for digestion including the stomach, intestines, liver and pancreas.

Keyword: Anatomy

Digital radiography
This method of taking an x-ray produces an image which can
be scanned within seconds and appears on a monitor and
is stored on a computer using specialised software. A sensor and
an x-ray holder are used to produce an instant image. Alterna-
tively a special reusable x-ray film is used with a holder which is
placed into a scanner and an image is produced in less than a
minute.

Keyword: Radiography

Disclosing agents
A topical solution or chewed tablet which will dye the teeth to
detect any plaque present. This reveals the invisible first forma-
tions of plaque. Once the patient can see where it is situated, it

encourages better brushing and prevents the plaque from thickening.

Keyword: Prevention of oral disease

Discoloured film

Developed x-rays can appear discoloured or smudged for several reasons: during manual processing solution can be contaminated, fixing is incomplete, it was not immersed fully in fixer, or it was washed inadequately after fixing.

Keyword: Radiography

Disinfection

Many products available that kill or prevent the growth of micro-organisms. Used when items and equipment can not be sterilised in an autoclave. Used also to clean surfaces. Some products can be used internally in dental procedures such as root canal treatment.

Keyword: Cross-infection control

Dislocation

The two bones in a joint become completely displaced and there is no contact. If this happens in the jaw it means that the condyle has slipped too far forward in front of the articular eminence and is stuck.

Keyword: Anatomy

Dispensing wells

These are used to hold materials such as bond and etch and passed to the operator so they can pick up the material on a brush for placing on the tooth. They are available in various shapes and sizes, and are disposable or sterilised.

Keyword: Restoration

Display screen equipment (DSE)

This term refers to computers and accessories used in the workplace. There is a Display Screen Equipment Act 1992 which will determine the persons in the work place who are deemed to be users of DSE. The Act provides guidelines to follow to protect users from injury or ill health as a result of improper use. Regular rest periods, suitable viewing position, good posture to prevent neck and back problems and foot rests are all among the recommended guidelines.

Keyword: Health and safety

Disposable cap
Worn by surgical staff and patient to isolate the head from the sterile operating area. Single use only.

Keyword: Cross-infection control

Dissecting forceps
A surgical instrument used by the operator to grasp soft tissue, keeping it taut whilst suturing is being done.

Keyword: Minor oral surgery

Distal end cutter
Used mainly to cut archwire during an orthodontic procedure before or after the wire is placed in the mouth. The archwire is held by the cutters so it does not fall into the patient's mouth. Available in various angles and sizes.

Keyword: Orthodontics

Distal tooth surface
This is the surface of the tooth which is furthest away from the midline of the arch facing towards the back of the tooth.

Keyword: Anatomy

DMF count
Decayed, missing and filled teeth. A public health survey comparing populations of areas that have different amounts of fluoride in the water supply.

Keyword: Prevention of dental disease

Dosimeter
A radiation monitoring badge worn by an individual in the surgery to measure the level of radiation received over a set period of time. Worn around the hip area and sent to the radiological board to read the levels. Usually only worn if a certain amount of radiographs are to be taken on a daily basis. The appointed radiation protection advisor (RPA) in the practice will have guidelines to follow.

Keyword: Radiography

Dovetail joint
This joint is incorporated between two parts of a fixed removable bridge to allow for slight flexibility.

Keyword: Prosthetic

Dry aid
See Dryguard

Keyword: Moisture control

Dryguard
These discs help control moisture during procedures such as a fillings. The absorbent material is placed over the parotid salivary gland duct and soaks up any saliva.

Keyword: Moisture control

Dry socket
This occurs when a blood clot fails to form in the socket of a recently extracted tooth. This can cause an infection or the tooth may have been infected before. This causes pain and a bad taste. The dry socket can be syringed with an antiseptic solution to remove debris. Painkillers are advised and a sedative dressing can be placed. In some cases, antibiotics are prescribed.

Keyword: Extraction/minor oral surgery

Dual curing resins
A luting cement which is a combination of self- and light-curing resins.

Keyword: Restorations/prosthetic

Duodenum
This is the first part of the small intestine extending from the stomach and part of the digestion process. It is about 25 cm long and loops around the head of the pancreas. Digestive enzymes and chemicals in the bile are released via a duct into the pancreas, liver and gall bladder.

Keyword: Digestion

Edentulous

This condition refers to a person who has no natural teeth.

Keyword: Anatomy

Elastic separators

Used during orthodontic procedures, they are placed in between teeth to create an interproximal space for bands to be placed soon after.

Keyword: Orthodontics

Elastomer

An impression material available in different types such as silicones and polyether. The base and the catalyst are mixed together and loaded into an impression tray for construction of a crown, bridge, inlay or veneer.

Keyword: Restorations/prosthetic

Electricity at Work Regulations (1989)

This is concerned with the safety of fixed and portable electrical appliances, including equipment that has a cable, a plug and is normally moved around such as kettles, lamps and printers. The supply to electrical appliances should be installed, wired and fused by registered contractors. The HSE has advised that dental practices have equipment tested every two to three years.

Keyword: Health and safety

Electric motor

This is an expensive piece of equipment that you will find on the dental unit. Handpieces are attached to it and it can reach speeds of 100,000 rpm.

Keyword: Handpieces and burs

Electric pulp tester
This piece of equipment enables a vitality test to be carried out on a tooth to determine whether the tooth is alive (vital) or dead (non-vital). An attachment is placed on the tooth and electronic stimulus is increased gradually until the patient can feel it indicating vitality.

Keyword: Endodontic

Elongation
This describes an exposure fault that can occur due to an operating error whilst taking a radiographic x-ray. The image on the film will appear long and runs off the film indicating the angle was too shallow.

Keyword: Radiography

E

Enamel
This is the hard outer layer of the tooth that covers and protects its inner structures. This substance is harder than bone and can not feel pain or sensitivity as it does not contain nerves or blood vessels.

Keyword: Anatomy

Enamel chisel
A double-ended instrument that comes in various shapes and sizes. Its working ends have sharp bevels to remove any enamel that is unsupported whilst preparing a cavity.

Keyword: Restoration

Enamel fluorosis
This condition can occur at the stage of the enamel formation if too much fluoride is ingested. Mottled white areas can be seen on the erupted enamel surface.

Keyword: Oral disease

Enamel hatchet
Same function as an enamel chisel. A double-ended instrument available in various shapes and sizes and removes unsupported enamel whilst preparing a cavity.

Keyword: Restoration

Endocrine system

This is a collection of glands that produce hormones including the thyroid gland, pancreas, testes, ovaries and adrenal glands. The endocrine system regulates and co-ordinates body workings such as growth and metabolism.

Keyword: Anatomy

Endodontics

The most common endodontic procedure carried out is root canal treatment. The term is used to describe a branch of dentistry that treats disease and injury affecting the nerves and pulp. Other treatments include pulpotomy, pulp capping and apicectomy.

Keyword: Endodontic

Endodontic block

Holds and organises filing instruments during root canal procedures and it has a measuring device incorporated. The block can be sterilised in the autoclave.

Keyword:-Endodontic

Endodontic handpiece

Used during root canal procedures and when using special rotary files. The handpiece has an adjustable speed which enables files to clean and shape the root canal.

Keyword: Endodontic

Endodontic K files

Different lengths are available and the sizes are colour coded. Each canal is cleaned and shaped by this file and the operator will increase the size of the file to enlarge the canal. These files are disposed of in the sharps container after use.

Keyword: Endodontic

Endodontic plugger

Used during root canal procedures to condense and pack the gutta percha root filling material, after it has been heated, in to the root canal.

Keywords: Endodontic

Endodontic ruler
Available as a metal ruler or incorporated on endodontic rings, blocks or the side of a treatment tray. Used to measure the lengths of files.

Keyword: Endodontic

Endospores
Found in bacteria and have a tough protective coating making them highly resistant. Spores found in the mouth are associated with chronic periodontal disease.

Keyword: Periodontal

Environmental Protection Act 1990
This act ensures that dental practices dispose of waste correctly and maintain records and documents relating to waste arrangements and collections by registered companies.

Keyword: Waste disposal/health and safety

Enzymes
There are thousands of enzymes in the body; each one has a different function. An enzyme is a protein made by the body that regulates the role of a chemical reaction in the body.

Keyword: Anatomy

Epiglottis
This is the visible flap of cartilage lying beneath the tongue which allows air to pass through the larynx and into the rest of the respiratory system. It also prevents food entering the larynx during swallowing.

Keyword: Anatomy

Epinephrine
Also known as adrenaline. A drug used to arrest haemorrhage by constricting bleeding capillaries. Applied externally as a solution.

Keyword: Drugs

Ergonomics
This means that the working environment is suitable for the worker, taking into account body size and shape, fitness and

strength, posture, senses, stresses on joints and muscles and psychological aspects of an individual. Ergonomics in the workplace can improve health and safety. In dentistry seating is very important, as is posture and positioning. An ergonomically sound working environment has to be present in order for the team to function together, especially in four-handed dentistry.

Keyword: Health and safety

Erosion
The loss of enamel from the tooth's surface. This can be caused by plaque, acids from certain food and drinks, vomiting and over brushing. Symptoms are sensitivity to hot, cold and sweet things.

Keyword: Oral disease

Eruption
This is the development of new teeth moving upwards through the jaw bone and breaking through the gum.

Keyword: Anatomy

Erythrocytes
Also known as red blood cells or red corpuscles. Their purpose is the transportation of oxygen and carbon dioxide between the lungs and all of the tissues of the body.

Keyword: Blood

Erythromycin
An antibiotic drug used to treat infections and prescribed to a patient who has a penicillin allergy.

Keyword: Drugs

Excavator
A double-ended instrument available in various sizes. Looks like a tiny spoon and is used to remove carious dentine.

Keyword: Restoration

Excretion
This simply means the discharge of waste material from the body including excess water and by-products of digestion. The kidneys,

liver, large intestine, lungs and sweat glands all discharge waste from the body.

Keyword: Digestion

Expansion screw

This is contained within an orthodontic appliance that is used to correct cross bites. By using a key, the screw is turned as instructed at regular intervals.

Keyword: Orthodontics

External respiration

This is the exchange of oxygen and carbon dioxide which occurs in the alveoli. From here, the oxygen passes from the lungs into the capillaries and carbon dioxide from the capillaries into the lungs.

Keyword: Anatomy

External verifier (EV)

This person is employed by an awarding body, such as City & Guilds, as an objective expert. The EV will monitor assessment and IV practices of approved training centres to ensure consistency and reliability of training decisions and to maintain quality standards set out for qualifications. The EV will conduct visits to approved training centres and give approval and verification of work undertaken by assessors and IVs.

Keyword: Training

Extraction

This is the removal of tooth/teeth by a dentist for reasons such as abscess, pain, periodontal disease, overcrowding, unrestorable or severely decayed. The procedure can be carried out under local anaesthetic or general anaesthetic.

Keyword: Extraction/minor oral surgery

Extra-oral

This means the soft tissues and joints outside of the oral cavity. These are checked during an extra-oral soft tissue assessment and include the lips, lymph nodes, moles, blemishes and facial symmetry.

Keyword: Anatomy

Extra-oral radiographs

Extra-oral means outside of the mouth. This type of panoramic x-ray film is placed inside a cassette and placed in a panoramic x-ray machine. The cassette containing the film moves all around the patient's head and produces a full view image of the mouth including joints and sinuses.

Keyword: Radiography

Extra-oral x-ray machine

Used for exposing radiographs that can be taken outside of the mouth, for example panoramic or cephalometric x-rays. The machine moves the x-ray all around the patient's head.

Keyword: Radiography

E

External oblique line

This is the faint ridge marking the base of the alveolar process of the body of the mandible and carries on behind the front border of the ramus.

Keyword: Anatomy

Eye protection

A full face visor or protective glasses should be worn during all clinical procedures. Glasses should be given to the patient as well. Full lenses are required to give full protection against splatter and particles. Visor screens should be changed regularly and glasses cleaned with correct detergents after every use.

Keyword: Health and safety

F

Face mask
Personal protective equipment (PPE) worn by operators to prevent splatter from blood, saliva, debris and micro-organisms from entering the eyes, mouth and nose.

Keyword: Health and safety

Face shield/visor
Personal protective equipment (PPE) worn by operators to prevent splatter from blood, saliva, debris and micro-organisms from entering the eyes, mouth and nose. They come as glasses and have a mask already attached to them or a see-through barrier is clipped to the ear arms and covers the whole face.

Keyword: Health and safety

Facial nerve
This is the 7th cranial nerve and arises from the structures in the brain stem performing motor and sensory functions. These control the muscles of the neck, facial expression, salivary glands and outer ear.

Keyword: Anatomy

Facial palsy
Inflammation or damage to the facial nerve causing weakness to the facial muscle. Can be temporary and affects one side of the face. It can come on suddenly and usually clears without treatment. In rare cases, treatment is required. Injury, herpes or a tumour can lead to this condition.

Keyword: Illness

Fainting
A form of collapse resulting in temporary loss of consciousness due to reduced blood flow to the brain. If a person falls down, then the legs can be raised restoring blood flow back to the brain; recovery can occur in minutes.

Keyword: Collapse/medical emergency

False pocket
This is formed when the gingiva is swollen, inflamed and red. The chronic gingiva forms a false pocket around the neck of the teeth allowing more plaque to develop below the margin.

Keyword: Oral disease

Fast handpiece
Also known as an air turbine, high speed and air rotor. Used during the preparation of restorations, fixed prosthetic appliances, shaping and polishing restorations using friction grip burs. It uses water and can run up to 500,000 rpm.

Keyword: Handpieces and burs

F

Fat
Fat is present in meat, fish, dairy products and oils providing the body with energy and body fat. The amount of fat in the body needs to be controlled. Saturated fat in large amounts is dangerous and can lead to a risk of heart disease. Some essential fatty acids are stored in the body for energy reserves and provide insulation.

Keyword: Digestion

Felypressin
A local anaesthetic drug used in conjunction with 3% prilocaine providing a longer lasting numbing action without having to use adrenalin.

Keyword: Local anaesthetic/drugs

Figure of eight calipers
A measuring device used to measure the thickness of porcelain and metal whilst constructing the prosthesis.

Keyword: Prosthetic and measuring devices

Filling
A restorative procedure that is carried out if a tooth has been chipped, fractured or decay has occurred. There are various types of filling material that can be used and they can be temporary or permanent depending on the treatment required.

Keyword: Restoration

Film holder
Used to hold an x-ray film when taking an intra-oral radiograph. Various ones are used depending on view of the tooth/teeth required and the nature of the treatment. Anterior peri-apical holders, posterior peri-apical holder, bitewing holder and endodontic holders all help towards ensuring a more accurate x-ray.

Keyword: Radiography

Finger spreader
A small hand instrument used during endodontic procedures to condense gutta percha filling material into the root canal during obturation (heating). They come in different sizes and are colour coded.

Keyword: Endodontic

Finishing strip
Used for polishing the interproximal surface of composite fillings. They vary in abrasiveness and can be used to remove stains from the tooth surface.

Keyword: Restoration

Fire Precaution Regulations 1997
This requires the practice to have a fire risk assessment carried out. The regulations specify that emergency routes and exits are to be kept free from obstruction at all times ensuring a quick and safe evacuation. Exits should lead to a place of safety and be clearly indicated. Emergency lighting should be provided where necessary and emergency doors must open in the direction of escape. Practices should have suitable fire fighting equipment as recommended.

Keyword: Health and safety

First aid box

All dental practices must have at least one first aid box which can be easily located, kept stocked and expiry dates checked. Items included should be: guidance leaflet on first aid, 20 individually wrapped sterile adhesive dressings, 2 sterile eye pads, 4 individually wrapped sterile bandages, 6 safety pins, 6 medium sized individually wrapped wound dressings, pair of disposable gloves, sterile water, saline or an eye wash solution.

Keyword: Health and safety

Fish-tail spatula

The mixing end is shaped like a fish tail and is used whilst mixing alginate impression material enabling the mixture to be spread inside the surface area of the bowl to produce a smooth mix.

Keyword: Prosthetics

F

Fissure

These are crevices in the occlusal tooth surfaces of the pre-molars and molars, between the cusps. They can be a stagnation area for plaque.

Keyword: Anatomy

Fissure sealant

Material used to fill crevices on the tooth surface, called fissures. The fluoride material is placed and it flows into the fissures and is set by the use of an ultraviolet light. This can prevent occlusal caries. Mainly done in children when molar teeth are erupting.

Keyword: Restoration

Fistula

This is an abnormal passage or perforation from an internal organ to the body's surface. It can also occur between two organs. In the mouth an oro-antral fistula can occur between the oral cavity and maxillary sinus. On rare occasions this can happen during an extraction which will need to be closed by suturing.

Keyword: Extraction/minor oral surgery

Fixed orthodontic appliance

Worn by an individual to correct their specific form of malocclusion or to reposition teeth. Brackets are cemented to the teeth and wire is passed through them and secured. They are tightened, applying pressure to the teeth to move them gradually over a period of time. The appliance is removed once the repositioning has been achieved and a retainer is worn to maintain the positioning of the teeth. Patients have different requirements and appliances are tailored to meet the needs of the individual.

Keyword: Orthodontic

Fixed prosthetic appliance
This refers to any laboratory made appliances such as crowns, bridges, inlays, veneers and implants that are fixed into the oral cavity either by cementation or retained within the root or bone.

Keyword: Prosthetic

Fixer
A solution used whilst developing an x-ray film. Measured in the correct quantity and used in a Velopex machine or in manual processing. The image is fixed onto the film at this stage of the processing and needs to be immersed in the solution for a certain amount of time.

Keyword: Radiography

Flat plastic
An instrument used mainly during filling procedures to place material into the cavity preparation. It is also used to remove excess material. Comes in various shapes, sizes and makes.

Keyword: Restoration

Flat ridge
The alveolar ridge can become flat over a period of time due to teeth being lost and the bone shrinking. This can be a problem especially on the lower ridge when a denture is worn. A patient can find this very difficult as there is not much bone to keep a lower denture in place, it will be loose and move about during speech and eating. A ridge can be built up by adding bone substitute to increase natural retention.

Keyword: Prosthetic

Floss
Required for interdental cleaning, removing plaque and food from in between the teeth. Available in thread or tape, waxed or unwaxed.

Keyword: Prevention of oral disease

Fluorapatite
These are crystals formed by the enamel when it has reminer-alised after an acid attack. This is done by exchanging fluoride to form fluorapatite crystals making the enamel surface harder and prepared for more acid attacks.

Keyword: Anatomy

Fluoride
A mineral that helps to prevent dental caries and strengthens the enamel surface. It can be naturally present in water, if not it can be added to local water systems depending on the council. Others ways of getting fluoride are by using a fluoride mouth-wash or toothpaste, supplements or as a topical application in the form of a gel. This makes the enamel more resistant to acid attacks.

Keyword: Prevention of dental disease

Fluorosis
Fluorosis of the enamel means that excessive amounts of fluoride have been ingested whilst the enamel was forming. This presents with teeth having noticeable mottled white areas and depending on the severity can be unsightly resulting in the need for cosmetic treatment.

Keyword: Oral conditions

Fogged film
An x-ray film may appear too dark or too grey as a result of being exposed to light before it is placed in fixer. The dark room must have no light intrusion. Another cause of fogged films is if they are stored in hot, humid environments, if they have expired or are stored too close to an x-ray set.

Keyword: Radiography

Foramen
This is an opening or hole in a bone or body structure allowing nerves and blood vessels to pass through. Foramens associated with dentistry are: apical, greater palatine, incisive, infra-orbital, magnum, mandibular and mental. These natural holes are in the base of the skull and nerves supplying the jaws, teeth and face exit the brain through here.

Keyword: Anatomy

Forceps
Various types of these tweezers-like instruments available for removing teeth, bone, roots and the handling of tissue. Each one is designed for a specific purpose.

Keyword: Extraction/minor oral surgery

Foreshortening
This is an exposure fault which can occur whilst taking an x-ray. The x-ray image will appear small and squashed due to the angulation of the x-ray tube being too steep.

Keyword: Radiography

Fox's occlusal plane guide
A device used whilst constructing a set of dentures for patients who have no teeth at all. Used at the bite registration stage, it checks the jaw relationship and determines the correct positioning of the teeth before they are set on the wax denture at the try-in stage.

Keyword: Prosthetics

Frenectomy
This means the removal of the frenum. The lingual frenum can restrict movement of the tongue and the upper labial frenum can cause a large gap to occur between the central incisors if too large. A surgical procedure is carried out to remove the fibrous tissue concerned.

Keyword: Minor oral surgery

Frenum
Thin bands of fibrous tissue; there are two situated in the oral cavity: under the upper lip and attached to the gum between the

incisors, and the lingual frenum at the floor of the mouth attached to the tongue.

Keyword: Anatomy

Friction grip bur

This is used in the air turbine for cutting into the tooth surface or on already restored teeth. They are made from tungsten carbide or diamond and are used to prepare cavities and fixed prosthetic appliances.

Keyword: Restoration/prosthetics

Fructose

A naturally occurring, simple sugar found in many foods, such as fruits and vegetables, which the body can use as energy. It does not cause blood sugars to rise but should still be taken in small amounts.

Keyword: Digestion

Functional orthodontic appliance

A removable orthodontic appliance made from acrylic and stainless steel designed to the requirements of the individual. This is worn in the upper and lower jaws at the same time and will correct malocclusion.

Keyword: Orthodontic

Full denture

Full upper, full lower or full set. A removable prosthetic appliance consisting of artificial replacement teeth. Worn to replace missing teeth and is made from acrylic.

Keyword: Prosthetic

Fungi

There are various forms of fungi, the harmful ones cause disease and illness. They are parasitic life forms larger than bacteria and are responsible for oral diseases such as, candida, denture stomatitis and thrush.

Keyword: Microbiology

Furcation

This is where the root of the tooth is divided and there is a loss of periodontal ligament. Furcation involvement is measured during a periodontal assessment when probing pocket depth measurements are recorded and graded using a special probe with measurement markings on it.

Keyword: Periodontal

F

G

Gall bladder
This stores bile which is produced in the liver until the body needs it for digestion. This pear-shaped sac is located under the liver.

Keyword: Anatomy

Gally pot
Comes in various sizes and is used to hold sterile saline solution for irrigation. Can also be used to drop dirty burs and other small instruments into to keep safe.

Keyword: Accessories

Gas cylinders
These supply a gas supply to bunsen burners that are used during the construction of prosthetic appliances. Most of these cylinders are stored in the practice and should be kept in a fire resistant place with adequate ventilation through to an external wall. These have a three-year shelf life and should be stored away from sources of ignition. Other gas cylinders include medical oxygen cylinders.

Keyword: Health and safety

Gates-Glidden burs
Used during endodontic procedures to remove previous root filling material from the root canal if the tooth is being prepared for a post crown. They are also used to gain access to the root canal by drilling into the pulp chamber. They are available in different sizes indicated by the number of rings located at the

opposite end and are latch grip. They are flame-shaped and disposed of in the sharps container.

Keyword: Endodontic

General anaesthetic
GA is carried out once a patient is unconscious after receiving intravenous anaesthetic to relax and paralyse the muscles. GA is done in hospital with a specially trained team. For dental treatment this is done as a last resort and only if the patient is a suitable candidate, with a clear medical history. The anaesthetic mixture is administered directly into the lungs through a nasotracheal tube passing through the nostrils, nasopharynx, larynx and trachea entering the airway. The patient will need to be monitored in recovery for a while until the GA has worn off.

Keyword: Sedation

General Dental Council (GDC)
This is the governing body of the dental profession. All dental care professionals from July 2008 will have to be registered with the council. Continuing professional development (CPD) is required and will have to be recorded and high standards of practice and conduct maintained at all times.

G

Keyword: Governing body

Gerontology
This is the study of ageing. Oral tissues, skin, bone, salivary glands and teeth will change with age and this is relevant when prescribing dental treatment to an older individual.

Keyword: Oral health

Gingiva
This is the Latin name for gums, which fit around the neck of each tooth protecting underlying structures. Healthy gums should appear pink and firm.

Keyword: Anatomy

Gingival crevice
This is the crevice between the tooth surface and gum margin. The crevice can be measured with a special measuring probe to

determine whether it is healthy or not. The measurements should be 3 mm or less.

Keyword: Anatomy

Gingival margin trimmer
Double-ended instrument with sharp bevelled working ends used to remove unsupported enamel whilst preparing a cavity.

Keyword: Restoration

Gingival retraction cord
Available in different thicknesses and pushed into the gingival crevice during a crown preparation procedure, retracting the gingiva so an accurate impression can be taken. The permanent prosthesis will fit perfectly to the gum margin when cemented.

Keyword: Prosthetic/restoration

Gingival retraction cord instrument
Also called a cord packer. Looks like a large excavator but has serrated edges and packs retraction cord into the gingival crevice.

Keyword: Prosthetic/restoration

Gingivectomy
This is the surgical removal of part of the gum margin. This is done due to excessive gum overgrowth or to remove pockets of infected gum.

Keyword: Periodontal disease

Gingivectomy knives
Used to remove the gingival tissue that has overgrown the natural margin. They are double ended instruments used in periodontal surgery. The different types are: Buck, Kirkland, Orban and Goldman-Fox.

Keyword: Minor oral surgery

Gingivoplasty
Similar to gingivectomy whereby gingival tissue is removed.

Keyword: Minor oral surgery

Glass ionomer cement
Consists of a powder containing alumino-silicates and liquid containing polyacrylic acid which are mixed together and used for lining a cavity, temporary fillings, small fillings, fillings in deciduous teeth and as an adhesive cement and fissure sealing.

Keyword: Restoration

Glenoid fossa (or mandibular fossa)
This is a hollow in the temporal bone and when the mouth is closed the condyle rests in this hollow.

Keyword: Anatomy

Glossopharyngeal nerve
This is the 9th cranial nerve performing motor and sensory functions. It supplies the parotid salivary glands, and regulates the secretion of saliva. It supplies taste sensation and controls the movement of throat muscles.

Keyword: Anatomy

G

Gloves
Gloves worn in the dental practice are single use only and should be worn for all clinical procedures. This form of personal protective equipment (PPE) protects against, blood, saliva and other body fluids. They play a very important role in cross-infection control and health and safety. Latex gloves are available, but most practices are now using vinyl due to an increase in latex allergy and dermatitis. Heavy duty gloves should be worn when scrubbing instruments and when handling potentially harmful chemicals.

Keyword: Cross-infection control/Health and safety

Glucose
A simple sugar that is naturally occurring in fruit and vegetables and provides energy for the body. Glucose is carried to all tissues in the blood stream, so levels should be constant. A high glucose level can result in hyperglycaemia; low levels in hypoglycaemia.

Keyword: Digestion

Glyceryl trinitrate (GTN)
This spray is found in the medical drugs kit and is used by patients who suffer from angina pain.

Keyword: Drugs

Gracey curettes
Many types and sizes available. Double-ended instruments, one end for cutting and the other rounded, usually comes in a set. Used in periodontal procedures to remove stains and calculus.

Keyword: Periodontal

Granulation tissue
This is a temporary repair tissue that develops on the surface of damaged or inflamed area of gum helping with the healing process. White cells and capillaries form scaffolding and reconstruct the damage.

Keyword: Pathology

Greater palatine nerve
This provides nerve supply to the distal half of the first molar, second and third molars including their buccal gingiva.

Keyword: Anatomy

Green occlusal indicating wax
Used to check the jaw relationship whilst assessing the bite or when fixing prosthetic appliances.

Keyword: Prosthetic

Green stick composition
This is heated with hot water and softened and used to adapt a standard impression tray to fit a patient's mouth better. The edges of the tray can be extended using this wax.

Keyword: Prosthetic

Guedel airway
Also known as the oropharyngeal airway. It is part of the emergency and oxygen kit and is used to keep an open airway and to prevent the patient's tongue falling back and blocking the airway.

Keyword: Collapse/emergencies

Guide drill

This is the first drill in the kit; it is a medium-round tungsten carbide on a long shank and is used to mark the site of implant placement and to perforate through the cortical bone into the cancellous bone. It may also be used to determine the direction of the implant.

Keyword: Implant

Gutta percha

Material used in a root filling procedure. This permanent filling is inserted into the clean dry root canal sealing the apical end of the canal. Used in conjunction with a cement and instrument that condenses the filling firmly providing a leak-proof seal.

Keyword: Endodontic

G

H

Haemoglobin
This is the oxygen-carrying pigment that is present in red blood cells which is produced by bone marrow and contains iron.

Keyword: Orthodontic

Haemophilia
An inherited blood clotting disorder. The blood clotting protein from the blood is deficient which may result in excessive bleeding that may be difficult to stop after injury or dental treatment.

Keyword: Pathology

Haemorrhage
Excessive bleeding which may be due to a condition called haemophilia or by the cutting of the blood vessels during surgical procedures.

Keyword: Pathology

Haemostasis
Meaning the arrest of bleeding. After an extraction a patient can leave the surgery once this has been achieved: the socket will stop bleeding because the small vessels constrict, blood cells plug the bleeding points, and plasma-forming fibrin seals the damaged vessel.

Keyword: Extractions/minor oral surgery

Haemostatic
These are drugs also known as styptics, used to treat bleeding disorders and control bleeding, for example adrenaline solution. This also applies to achieving haemostasis after an extraction by means of clotting agents packed into the socket such as Kaltostat

or by means of a bite pack or gauze placed over the socket for a few minutes until a blood clot has formed.

Keyword: Drugs

Halitosis
Bad breath caused by smoking, drinking alcohol, eating strong tasting foods, poor hygiene or stomach-related problems.

Keyword: Oral health promotion

Hand file
Small instrument used during endodontic procedures. Available in different lengths and are colour coded. Used as a hand instrument to shape and enlarge a root canal. These are single use only and disposed of in sharps container.

Keyword: Endodontic

Hand washing instruments
This method of cleaning instruments prior to sterilisation must be done with care following recommended guidelines to avoid inoculation injuries. The instruments should be immersed in a sink of tepid water and detergent and when scrubbing using a long-handled brush, brush away from the body. Brushes are available that can be sterilised in the autoclave and this should be done at regular intervals.

Keyword: Health and safety/Cross-infection control

H

Hard reline
Material can be added to an acrylic denture that is nearly at the end of its life to replace reabsorbed bone. This can be done in the surgery or sent to a laboratory. This will help the denture feel a little more secure and comfortable until a new one is made.

Keyword: Prosthetics

Hawe supermat matrix
Stainless steel and clear disposable matrices used for posterior composite and amalgam restorations. They come in different sizes in a kit and their function is to replace proximal walls around the tooth. A special instrument comes in the kit to help place the matrix.

Keyword: Restoration

Hazardous substance

A risk assessment will determine the substances used in the dental practice that could be potentially harmful. This is required under the COSHH Regulations. A hazardous substance can be harmful, corrosive, toxic or an irritant. A COSHH report will address the risk and specify measures in reducing or controlling the risk.

Keyword: Health and safety

Headgear and face bow

An orthodontic appliance worn to restrict the growth of the maxillary arch, preventing deep overbites. The headgear is worn outside the mouth and the inner bow is attached to the buccal tubes intra-orally.

Keyword: Orthodontic

Health and Safety at Work Act (1974)

A law designed to protect staff and patients by providing legislations and protocols for maintaining a safe working environment.

Keyword: Health and safety

Health and Safety Executive, The (HSE)

This statutory body is responsible for enforcing The Health and Safety at Work Act. It provides an advisory service and gives health and safety inspectors the power to enter premises to examine all areas of the practice. They can ask for information, interview and take written statements from anyone they think can help with their investigation. The inspectors are not legally bound to announce their visit but will normally make appointments. They inspect all equipment and electrical appliances, check reports, certificates and the practice's health and safety policy.

Keyword: Health and safety

Heart

A muscular pump sending blood to the lungs and the rest of the body. The heart is located in the centre of the chest and beats at an average 72 bpm. The heart divides into two upper chambers, right and left atriums, and two lower chambers, right and left ventricles. The upper and lower compartments are connected with valves.

Keyword: Heart and circulation

Heimlich manoeuvre
A first aid procedure used to remove lodged material that is causing a blockage in the airway. An abdominal thrust is performed by a first aider, placing their fists under the individual's rib cage and pulling inwards and upwards.

Keyword: First aid/emergency procedures

Hepatitis B virus (HBV)
A disease that is transmitted in blood or other body fluids. The incubation period is one to six months. The disease infects the liver, causing inflammation and symptoms such as headache, fever and jaundice. Some people are undiagnosed (carriers) due to very mild symptoms and others result in liver cancers. Vaccinations are available to healthcare workers and other workers who may be at risk of exposure.

Keyword: Pathology

Hepatitis C virus (HCV)
Very similar to hepatitis B and is transmitted by blood-blood contact from an infectious person. HCV has a high mortality rate and there is no vaccination available. The incubation period is six to twelve months and symptoms can progress to cirrhosis of the liver.

Keyword: Pathology

Herpes
An infection caused by the herpes simplex virus, usually characterised by the appearance of small blisters or cold sores on the skin, which may be painful. The virus is very contagious and is spread by direct contact.

Keyword: Pathology

High volume suction tip
Comes in various sizes and most are single use, though metal ones are still used and are autoclavable. Used to aspirate saliva,

blood and debris from the patient's mouth during clinical procedures. They can retract and protect soft tissues allowing the operator to have a clear field of vision.

Keyword: Moisture control

Hobson plugger
A double-ended filling instrument used to pack and condense amalgam into the cavity. Comes in various sizes and has two flat working ends.

Keyword: Fillings/restorative

Hoe
Used during periodontal procedures, can be single- or double-ended and different types are available. They remove supra- and sub-gingival calculus and plaque.

Keyword: Periodontal

Hormone
A chemical that is released by glands into the bloodstream or tissues to carry information and control many body functions such as growth.

Keyword: Anatomy/pathology

Horizontal impaction
This describes a tooth that is lying on its side which can be facing mesially or distally or across the dental ridge.

Keyword: Anatomy

Howe pliers
Orthodontic pliers used to grasp bands and archwire during cementation or removal of an orthodontic appliance. The long beak varies in size and shape.

Keyword: Orthodontic

Hydrocortisone
Produced naturally by the adrenal glands to regulate body functions and respond to changes such as stress, blood pressure and blood sugar levels. It is also synthetically produced and prescribed as a drug to replace this chemical if the body does not make enough. It is used to treat allergies and inflammation.

Keyword: Drugs

Hydrogen peroxide
An antiseptic irrigation solution used to treat infections such as dry sockets. It can also be used as a cleansing mouthwash.

Keyword: Drugs

Hydroxyapatite
This calcium phosphate mineral is the crystal structure of the enamel. It is a major component of the teeth and the molecules form microscopic crystal clumps.

Keyword: Anatomy

Hygienist
A qualified, trained dental care professional who is instructed by a dentist to treat patients who require treatments such as scaling, fissure sealants, administration of local anaesthetic, oral health and toothbrush instruction, diet advice and application of fluoride.

Keyword: PCD/periodontal

Hyoid bone
This U-shaped bone is situated centrally in the upper part of the neck and is not articulated to any other bone. It is supported by muscles in the neck and supports the roof of the tongue.

Keyword: Anatomy

H

Hypertension
This is commonly referred to as high blood pressure.

Keyword: Medical condition

Hypodontia
This means naturally having fewer than the regular amount of teeth, most commonly missing are third molars and second premolars.

Keyword: Anatomy

Hypoglossal nerve
The 12th cranial nerve supplying movement to the tongue only.

Keyword: Anatomy

Hypoglycaemia
Meaning 'under sweet blood'. A condition caused by an abnormally low level of blood glucose not providing fuel to the brain.

This usually occurs in people who have diabetes. The symptoms can be sweating, hunger, dizziness, trembling, headaches, confusion, and double vision, and in severe cases a coma can occur. Insulin will need to be administered.

Keyword: Collapse

Hypoxia

Deprivation of oxygen to the body as a whole or a region of the body. This may be a result of strenuous exercise causing temperature hypoxia or in more serious cases, high altitude sickness, possibly leading to a pulmonary oedema. Symptoms are sickness, headaches, fatigue and impaired breathing.

Keyword: Collapse

H

Ibuprofen
An analgesic drug which is a non-steroidal, anti-inflammatory drug (NSAID) used as a painkiller and to reduce joint pain.

Keyword: Drugs

Identification rings
Coloured rings available in different types and sizes. They can be placed on instruments to identify and organise them. They can be sterilised.

Keyword: Accessories

Immediate replacement denture
An acrylic immediate denture can be made very quickly for patients who require an extraction. Once the tooth is removed the immediate denture with the missing tooth on it is placed in the mouth so that the patient is not left with an embarrassing gap. The impression for this type of denture is taken a day or two before the tooth is taken out.

Keyword: Prosthetic

Immune compromised
An individual with a compromised immune system is at risk from serious infections. For example, people who are HIV positive or who have cancer are immune compromised. The elderly can also be at risk and certain medications can reduce immune function.

Keyword: Pathology

Immunisation
This is a vaccine that will protect someone who is likely to come into direct contact with several serious, contagious diseases. In

dentistry, for example, staff are immunised against Hepatitis B. Most immunisations are given by injection and have no appreciable side effects.

Keyword: Infection control

Immunity
Resistance and protection to disease through the activity of the immune system. Certain white blood cells release antibodies and anti-toxins into the blood plasma.

Keyword: Pathology

Impaction
Failure of a tooth to fully erupt from the gum. This could be due to over crowding or a tooth growing in the wrong direction. Most commonly it is the lower wisdom teeth that are impacted and may require surgical extraction if they cause problems and regular infection.

Keyword: Minor oral surgery

Implants
Made of titanium and implanted into the alveolar bone. An implant is used as an artificial root where tooth/teeth are missing. The prosthetic structure will be placed on top of the implant once the healing process is complete. This will look and act as a natural tooth. The implant is drilled into the bone under sterile conditions using specialist implant instruments and equipment.

Keyword: Implants/minor oral surgery

Implant driver
Part of a dental implant kit. Available in two diameters and lengths to fit all implants. Looks like a long attachment drill.

Keyword: Implants

Implant kit
This kit contains specialist drills and instruments of varying types used for implant surgery. The drills have a specific place in the kit which is clearly marked making it easier to identify. There are various types and makes of kits available.

Keyword: Minor oral surgery

Implant scaler
The tips of the implant scaler are made from plastic or gold so as not to scratch or damage the implant whilst removing plaque or calculus build up from the implant area.

Keyword: Implants

Impression
Taken of the teeth to cast study models, enabling the construction of fixed and removable prosthetic appliances, orthodontic appliances, bleaching trays and diagnostic wax-ups. Many impression materials are available depending upon the treatment type. The material required is loaded into an impression tray and inserted into the oral cavity until set, providing a mould of the teeth, gums and bony ridges.

Keyword: Prosthetics

Impression decontamination
Once removed from the mouth, impressions should be rinsed to remove blood, saliva and any other debris. Once visibly clean they should be immersed in a disinfectant solution following manufacturer instructions. The impressions should be rinsed again and packaged appropriately. The practice should have an agreed impression disinfection policy with the laboratory. Lab tickets will have a box to indicate whether the impressions have been decontaminated.

Keyword: Cross-infection control

Impression paste
Sometimes called composition, made from zinc oxide eugenol and other constituents. One tube contains white zinc oxide and the other contains red eugenol. Equal quantities are mixed together with a plastic spatula to produce a suitable impression paste used as a wash or for relining loose dentures. The paste will be added to the acrylic and sent to the lab.

Keyword: Impression material

Incisal tooth surface
This is the biting edges of incisors and canines.

Keyword: Anatomy

Incisor
There are two central incisors at the front of the mouth and two lateral incisors either side of them. They each have a single root and a flattened biting edge.

Keyword: Anatomy

Index of Orthodontic Treatment Needs (IOTN)
A clinical assessment usually done during an exam whilst monitoring a patient's occlusion. The severity of the malocclusion is scored from 1–5 and if necessary is referred to an orthodontist for a second opinion and possibly for some form of orthodontic appliance to correct the problem.

Keyword: Orthodontics

Infection
This occurs in the body by disease-causing micro-organisms such as bacteria, fungi and viruses. These organisms reproduce and cause disease by damaging cells or by releasing toxins. Infection can cause symptoms such as aching joints or abscess, localised in a certain area of the body as a result of the body's immune system responding.

Keyword: Pathology

Infective endocarditis
People who have had congenital heart defects, a history of rheumatic fever or artificial heart valves are most at risk of this condition during procedures that may result in bacteria entering the patients' blood, for example extraction or scaling. The already damaged heart valves harbour these bacteria in the blood and provide protection from white cells. Infected clots of blood can spread throughout the body causing a very serious condition. As a preventive measure, all patients who are at risk are given antibiotic cover one hour prior to treatment.

Keyword: Pathology

Inferior alveolar nerve
Also known as the inferior dental nerve. This nerve supplies all the lower teeth.

Keyword: Drugs

Inferior dental block

Also known as ID nerve block. This injection of local anaesthetic solution anaesthetises the nerves in the soft tissue before it enters the lower jaw. It will numb several lower teeth, the lingual gum and half the tongue on the required side, as well as half the lower lip. The local anaesthetic is injected over the mandibular foramen anaesthetising the site of the inferior alveolar and lingual nerves.

Keyword: Local anaesthetic

Inferior dental nerve

A branch of the mandibular division. This nerve supplies all lower teeth, labial and buccal gingiva of the pre-molar, canine and incisors including soft tissues of the lower lip and the chin.

Keyword: Anatomy

Infiltration injection

A local anaesthetic that is given over the apex of the tooth and anaesthetises the nerve endings supplying the tooth and gum.

Keyword: Local anaesthetic

Inflammation

The symptoms present as redness, swelling, heat and pain present in a tissue as a result of injury or infection. Blood flow is increased to the damaged tissue and fluid leaks out of the capillaries causing localised swelling. The number of white blood cells increases causing inflammation and the pain is caused by stimulation of nerve endings.

Keyword: Pathology

Informed consent

Good communication will provide patients with full and detailed information regarding their treatment enabling them to give consent to proceed with the planned treatment.

Keyword: Communication

Inhalation sedation

Also known as relative anaesthesia (RA), this is used to sedate children under 16 years of age. It is a safe and efficient analgesic gas, a mixture of nitrous oxide (N_2O) and oxygen (O_2). The patient remains conscious, but does not feel pain as long as the gas is inhaled. Sometimes a local anaesthetic is also administered.

Keyword: Sedation

Injection
An injection used during dental procedures introduces a local anaesthetic solution into the body from a syringe via a needle to a localised area of the mouth. An injection can also be administered into a vein, muscle, joint or the skin.

Keyword: Local anaesthetic

Inlay
Used as an alternative to fillings, they are a fixed prosthesis made by a dental laboratory that will need to be cemented into the already prepared cavity of the tooth. They can be made from a gold, porcelain or composite material. The purpose of an inlay is to provide a stronger, more permanent restoration in a large cavity.

Keyword: Restoration

Inoculation injury
This occurs if a contaminated sharp instrument (e.g. a needle) has broken the surface of the skin or a substance (e.g. blood or saliva) has splashed in the eyes or onto a cut. This could also include a bite or scratch from a patient. Most common cause is from a needle after dismantling a local anaesthetic syringe.

Keyword: Health and safety/cross-infection control

Instrument cassettes
Can be used as an instrument tray or used to place instruments on during sterilisation for easy identification. Available in various sizes and make.

Keyword: Infection control

Insulin
Taken by people with diabetes to control their blood sugar level. The pancreas of diabetics does not produce this hormone, so an insulin replacement is administered.

Keyword: Drugs

Intensifying screens
Contained in an extra-oral film cassette. The screen increases the speed of the system, enabling the use of a lower dose of radiation. They absorb the x-ray and expose the film forming an image.

Keyword: Radiography

Interdental
Inter is a prefix meaning between, in dentistry this means in between the teeth.

Keyword: Anatomy

Internal verifier (IV)
This person supports and works with an NVQ assessor to develop assessment procedures and to facilitate good practice. The IV will work for awarding bodies, such as City & Guilds, and keep the assessor informed of new developments, techniques and training. The IV will sample pieces of evidence in trainee portfolios to monitor assessments recorded by the assessor. The role of the IV is to organise standardisation meetings to ensure that all assessors are working at an agreed level.

Keyword: Training

Intestine
Divided into two parts, small and large intestines. It is a major part of the digestive system extending from the exit of the stomach to the anus. (see Small intestine and Large intestine)

Keyword: Digestion

Intra-ligamentary syringes
A syringe with a short or ultra short needle and a small cartridge of local anaesthetic that delivers the solution into the periodontal ligament, directly through the gingival crevice. This is called an intra-ligamentary injection.

Keyword: Local anaesthetic

Intra-oral
This simply relates to anything contained inside of the oral cavity, for example the tongue or buccal mucosa. All of the intra-oral tissues are checked during a dental examination.

Keyword: Anatomy

Intra-oral camera

Used to show the dentist and patient the view from inside the oral cavity. This device is linked to dental software and will provide images on a monitor which can be saved in the patient's records. The camera magnifies the area of interest.

Keyword: Diagnosis

Intra-oral radiograph

These x-rays films produce images when exposed in the patient's mouth. X-rays taken inside the oral cavity include bitewings, periapicals and occlusal radiographs.

Keyword: Radiography

Intra-oral x-ray machine

This machine will vary depending on manufacturer. The tube of the machine is positioned overlying the film which has been placed inside the oral cavity, usually in a film holder exposing it. The machine is fixed on to the wall and the controls for the settings are positioned far enough away from the direct beam preventing exposure to unnecessary radiation, sometimes enabling the operator to stand outside of the room.

Keyword: Radiography

Intra-osseous injection

Used mainly when doing extractions, works immediately and provides a short duration of anaesthesia to the tooth. It is directly administered into the spongy bone between the tooth and gum only after the tooth has been anesthetised first. This will numb the tooth, the buccal and lingual gum.

Keyword: Local anaesthetic

Intravenous sedation

A tranquilliser is injected intravenously which relaxes the patient so the operator can administer a local anaesthetic and carry out the planned dental treatment. It produces amnesia while the drug is being administered so the patient will forget the procedure.

Keyword: Sedation

Iodine

Iodine compounds are used in dentistry as anaesthetics or for disinfecting an area before local anaesthetic is administered. It can also be used before an extraction to disinfect the gingival crevice.

Keyword: Drugs

Ionising Radiation Legislation (IRR 1999)

This regulation provides for the protection of staff and the public from the misuse or over use of x-rays. All dental practices must inform the Health and Safety Executive (HSE), who govern this legislation, of the use of routine x-ray equipment. Regular checks and services are carried out on all radiography equipment.

Keyword: Radiography

Ionising Radiation Medical Exposures Regulations 2000 (IRMER)

An IRMER practitioner, usually the dentist, takes responsibility for the regulation of exposure of individuals to potentially dangerous procedures, and ensures that the benefits of gaining diagnostic insight outweigh any potential hazards. Typical deciding factors before taking a radiograph include the frequency of previous radiographs, the reason and diagnostic benefit to the patient, and whether alternative techniques of diagnosis could be applied.

Keyword: Radiology

Iron

A mineral that is found in foods such as liver, nuts, fish and vegetables. It is essential for oxygen transport and cell growth. A lack of iron can result in little or no oxygen being delivered to cells, resulting in fatigue and anaemia. Iron supplements can be taken.

Keyword: Digestion

Irradiation

This is a method of sterilisation that exposes products to radiation. The exposure to gamma rays destroys micro-organisms, bacteria and viruses. This is an industrial process achieved by specialist equipment and can not be done in a dental surgery.

Keyword: Sterilisation/Cross-infection control

Irreversible pulpitis

This is caused by very deep caries lying close to the pulp or actually exposing it. The pulp at this stage will be very close to becoming non-vital (dead) if not already. The only methods of treating this are root canal treatment or an extraction.

Keyword: Endodontic

Irrigating syringe

Used with a disposable needle to irrigate and disinfect root canals and other infected areas of the mouth during endodontic procedures. The solution is delivered into the syringe and the sterile needle is placed at the end ready for use. The syringes are available in different sizes and are single use.

Keyword: Endodontic

Irrigation tubing set

This is attached to a saline polyfusor which attaches to the surgical handpiece providing sterile solution used to irrigate the site during surgical procedures, such as implants.

Keyword: Implant/minor oral surgery

Irritant

A substance can be classed as an irritant and cause irritation if not used correctly. The packaging will have a symbol warning of this potential hazard of skin inflammation, redness and dry skin, symptoms of contact dermatitis.

Keyword: Health and safety

Isolation

Isolation of a single tooth or teeth means that the operator can work on one or more teeth whilst being shielded from saliva and soft tissues. This is done by using rubber dam that provides moisture control allowing materials to set and protects the airway from inhalation of fluids or small instruments. Aspirating the area is made easier and can be done without the risk of harming soft tissues or causing burns.

Keyword: Moisture control

Iwanson gauge

Used for measuring the thickness of porcelain and metal during prosthetic procedures, mainly used in dental laboratories.

Keyword: Prosthetic/restoration

J

Jacquette scaler
A double- or single-handed instrument with sharp cutting edges used during periodontal procedures to remove supra-gingival calculus and plaque.

Keyword: Periodontal

Jaundice
There are different types of jaundice and all indicate disorders of the liver. Symptoms are yellowing of the skin and the whites of the eyes. This is caused by an accumulation of bilirubin in the blood which is formed from haemoglobin and absorbed by the liver. Sometimes, too much of this is produced for the liver to process.

Keyword: Pathology

Jaws
The upper jaw is called the maxilla and the lower is called the mandible. (see Mandible and Maxilla)

Keyword: Anatomy

Johnson contouring pliers
Used to contour and adapt an orthodontic band and stainless steel crown for placement on a tooth. This instrument has two beaks, one is used to secure the band or crown and the other one is used to contour.

Keyword: Restoration/orthodontics

K

Key skills
If a trainee nurse is working towards his or her NVQ Oral Health Care: Dental Nursing qualification and they do not possess GCSE grade C or above in Maths and English (or an equivalent qualification), they must complete Key Skills level II in Application of Number (AON) and Communication. These are recognised as GCSE grade C equivalent qualifications, and are useful and desirable skills for all aspects of work and life.

Keyword: Training

Kidney
The kidneys are situated at the back of the abdominal cavity on either side of the spine. They filter blood and excrete waste products such as urine from the body.

Keyword: Anatomy

Kidney dish
Used to hold instruments, liquids or materials during surgical procedures only if sterile. Can be used if a patient becomes ill or needs to spit into it after a rinse. They can be disposable or, if metal, can be sterilised in the autoclave.

Keyword: Minor oral surgery

Kilner cheek retractor
Retracts the cheek providing a clear field of vision for the operator mainly during surgical treatment.

Keyword: Minor oral surgery

L

Labial tooth surface
This is the tooth surface of the incisors and canines facing the cheeks.

Keyword: Anatomy

Lactobacillus
A rod-shaped bacteria, already present in the mouth, can be found in decayed teeth. They thrive in an acid environment enabling them to carry on the process of caries activity. Plaque that sticks to the teeth from food and debris in conjunction with these bacteria will start the decay process.

Keyword: Pathology

Lactose
A sugar found naturally in milk and is a good source of energy and helps the body to absorb minerals.

Keyword: Digestion

Lamina dura
This is the compact bone which lines the tooth socket. Any loss of this bone will indicate dental disease.

Keyword: Anatomy

Lancing
This is done to an abscess to release the infection. A tiny surgical incision is made to the abscess allowing the infection to drain.

Keyword: Pathology

Laryngoscope
This tube is part of a kit used in general anaesthesia. It is guided by direct vision through the larynx and into the trachea.

Keyword: Sedation

Larynx
Also known as the voice box. This organ in the throat is responsible for voice production. Its areas of cartilage project to form the Adam's Apple. It is situated between the pharynx and trachea.

Keyword: Anatomy

Laser scanner
Used during digital radiography. The scanner is set up to use with a computer that has digital x-ray software installed. The exposed sensor plate of the x-ray is inserted into the scanner and produces an image on the monitor in less than a minute.

Keyword: Radiography

Latch grip bur
This type of steel bur fits into a conventional handpiece. It comes in various sizes and shapes and is used for removing softened carious dentine. Other latch grip attachments are used for polishing.

Keyword: Burs and handpieces

Lateral condenser
Also known as finger spreader (see Finger spreader).

Keyword: Endodontic

Lateral periodontal abscess
An abscess which occurs on the side/laterally of the root of a vital tooth. This localised collection of pus needs to be drained and antibiotics will be prescribed.

Keyword: Pathology

Lateral pterygoid
This is a muscle of mastication allowing the mandible to be pulled forward by the pulling of joint cartilage; this aids in chewing.

Keyword: Anatomy

L

Lead apron
Used to protect patients from radiation whilst having an x-ray taken. The apron, along with a thyroid collar, gives protection to internal organs and tissues. There is no justification to use these with modern equipment. Lead aprons should be provided for pregnant patients and for the staff member who assists a child or disabled patient during radiography.

Keyword: Radiography

Le Cron carver
Used to trim the wax during the construction of a denture at the wax try-in or bite stages.

Keyword: Prosthetic

Leukaemia
A type of cancer affecting white blood cells within the bone marrow. Many organs can fail to function properly if they become affected by abnormal cells. In dentistry a patient with leukaemia will present with enlarged bleeding gums.

Keyword: Pathology

Leukocytes
Any type of white blood cell that protects the body against infection and fights it should an infection occur.

Keyword: Pathology

Lichen planus
A common skin disease, its cause is unknown. There are reasons to suggest that it can be brought on by stress. It presents as reddish, purplish bumps occurring anywhere on the skin. In the mouth it affects the inside of the cheeks, the gums and tongue. Oral lichen planus presents as white patches. Often a biopsy is carried out to confirm diagnosis.

Keyword: Pathology

Lidocaine
A local anaesthetic solution also known as lignocaine, it contains a small quantity of adrenaline to prolong the duration of the anaesthetic.

Keyword: Drugs/local anaesthetic

Ligature
Pre-shaped wire used to hold orthodontic archwire in place around the brackets on the teeth; it can be made from a variety of materials.

Keyword: Orthodontic

Ligature cutter
Used to cut ligature wire, elastic and power chains with its sharp edges during orthodontic procedures.

Keyword: Orthodontics

Ligature tucker
Single or double ended instrument used to tuck and bend ligature wire away from soft tissues to help prevent trauma to them.

Keyword: Orthodontics

Light reflecting wedges
These single-use items are used during the placement of a composite filling to reflect the light from the light curer onto the composite helping to set it. They are used with a matrix to help support it, maintain contact points and prevent ledges.

Keyword: Restoration

Light wire pliers
Used during orthodontic procedures to bend and create loops in archwire; different varieties are available.

Keyword: Orthodontics

Lingual frenum
This thin band of fibrous tissue attaches the tongue to the floor of the mouth.

Keyword: Anatomy

Lingual nerve
Situated in the mandibular division of the trigeminal nerve. This is one of the four branches that provide nerve supply to the lingual gingiva (floor of the mouth) of all lower teeth.

Keyword: Anatomy

L

Lingual tooth surface
This is the surface of all lower teeth facing the tongue and other lingual soft tissues.

Keyword: Anatomy

Lining
Many types of material available to line the cavity of a deep temporary or permanent filling. This means that the pulp will not be irritated and is protected from hot and cold of metal fillings.

Keyword: Restoration/linings

Liver
The largest organ of the body, it produces and processes a wide range of chemical substances including proteins for blood plasma. It produces cholesterol, secretes bile removing waste products, stores vitamins and breaks down fat.

Keyword: Anatomy/digestion

Local rules
The person in the practice, usually the dentist, who provides rules regarding radiation protection. These rules will be displayed in the practice and will show: the name of the radiation protection advisor (RPA) and radiation protection supervisor (RPS); designated controlled area; radiation dose levels; safety protocol; and information on what to do in case of equipment malfunction.

Keyword: Radiation

Localised osteitis
Inflammation of the bone commonly caused by infection. In dentistry it is called a dry socket. Bacteria present in the mouth attack the bone walls of the socket of a recently extracted tooth. If the blood clot has been lost, irrigation and antibiotics are required to treat this painful condition.

Keyword: Extraction

Long buccal nerve
A branch of the mandibular division providing nerve supply to the buccal gingiva of the lower molar teeth.

Keyword: Anatomy

Long shank surgical bur
Various shapes and sizes are available and it attaches into the straight handpiece to be used during surgical procedures for bone removal.

Keyword: Burs/handpieces

Low volume suction
A saliva ejector is usually placed into this part of the suction unit enabling a low volume removal of saliva that may collect in the patient's mouth during treatment. The ejector can stay in the patient's mouth throughout treatment to help with moisture control and to help retract the tongue.

Keyword: Moisture control

Lower deciduous anterior forceps
These forceps are used to remove lower deciduous teeth situated at the front of the mouth.

Keyword: Extractions

Lower deciduous molar forceps
Forceps used to remove lower deciduous teeth and also lower small permanent molars, right or left hand side.

Keyword: Extractions

Lower permanent pre-molar forceps
Used to extract lower permanent pre-molar teeth as well as anterior teeth, left or right side. The long thin beaks can also help to remove retained roots.

Keyword: Extractions

Lungs
Two main organs of the respiratory system supplying the body with oxygen. Air enters the lungs by the trachea branching off into the bronchus supplying each lung.

Keyword: Respiratory/anatomy

L

Luting cements
Different types of cement are available which adhere to the tooth tissue and inner surface of the prosthetic, either chemically or

mechanically. The prosthesis will be permanently fixed with this cement.

Keyword: Restoration

Luxator

A type of elevator used during difficult extractions to aid in the removal of roots and single-root teeth.

Keyword: Extraction/minor oral surgery

Lymph node

This small organ of tissue lies along lymphatic vessels associated with defence against infection. If the lymph node in the neck is swollen then this indicates infection. Lymph nodes are checked during an oral examination and if swollen, this can also indicate a tumour.

Keyword: Anatomy

L

M

Malignant
Heard when diagnosing a cancer or a tumour that can spread to nearby tissue or other parts of the body. A benign tumour means that it is non-cancerous.

Keyword: Pathology

Malocclusion
This is an abnormal relationship between the upper and lower set of permanent teeth when in the biting position. Orthodontic treatment will correct the malocclusion and teeth have a normal occlusion.

Keyword: Orthodontic

Mandible
This is what we refer to as the lower jaw. It is composed of two bones joining at mid-line. Its rotary movement allows the crushing of food in our mouths and its forward movement enables incisors to grasp food. Nerves and blood vessels that supply the teeth and soft tissues have passage ways through holes contained within the jaw.

Keyword: Anatomy

Mandrels
Discs are fitted to these latch-grip attachments in order to polish and smooth restorations. Various types are available.

Keyword: Restorations

Manual handling
The Manual Handling Operations Regulations 1992 provides clear duties for the employer and employee to protect against potential injuries. Manual handling should be avoided wherever

M

possible and if it can not be avoided then the risk should be assessed prior to handling, such as weight, environment and individual capacity.

Keyword: Health and safety

Marginal leakage
This can happen down the sides of a restoration. Microscopic gaps under the filling can mean that oral fluid can penetrate causing caries.

Keyword: Restorations

Mastication
Known as chewing, this is the first stage of digestion mixing broken down, chewed food with saliva.

Keyword: Digestion

Mathieu ligature pliers
The beaks of this orthodontic instrument grasp and place ligature wires and elastics whilst fitting or adjusting an orthodontic appliance. Its handle has a spring-loaded locking mechanism.

Keyword: Orthodontic

Mauns heavy duty wire cutters
Used mainly in orthodontic procedures to cut heavy excess archwire outside of the patient's mouth.

Keyword: Orthodontic

Maxilla
This is the upper jaw. A maxillary sinus is present left and right side. This sinus is a large air-filled cavity that is connected to the nasal cavity forming the hard palate. Nerves and blood vessels that supply the teeth and soft tissues have passage ways through holes contained in the jaw.

Keyword: Anatomy

Maxillary antrum
An air-filled cavity within the maxillary bones where various nerves and vessels are contained.

Keyword: Anatomy

M

Maxillary occlusal radiograph
This type of x-ray is taken in order to view any problems associated with upper incisors and their roots. The presence of supernumerary teeth can be detected and the image can determine the position of unerupted teeth.

Keyword: Radiography

Maxillary sinus
One of the largest paranasal sinuses forming a cavity in the floor of the maxilla. The upper pre-molars and molars are very close to this floor and care is taken not to perforate this floor of the sinus during an extraction of one of these teeth.

Keyword: Anatomy

Mayo needle holders
A surgical instrument that looks like a pair of scissors and is used during suturing. The suture is held firmly by the locking mechanism.

Keyword: Minor oral surgery

McKesson mouth prop
Used to keep the mouth propped open during surgery if the patient is struggling or uncomfortable. It is made of rubber and has a chain which is left extra-orally for safety reasons. The patient bites down on the prop on the opposite side of the mouth to where the operator is working, keeping the full mouth open.

Keyword: Instruments

Medial pterygoid
This is a muscle of mastication which enables the closing movement of the lower jaw.

Keyword: Anatomy

Megadont
These are abnormally large teeth that are erupting in a normal size jaw. The overcrowding will result in malocclusion.

Keyword: Orthodontic

M

Melanoma
An unusual blemish can indicate early signs of cancer, so the melanoma is investigated early. This can be done with a soft tissue exam.

Keyword: Examination/oral health

Mental nerve
A sensory nerve providing sensation to the buccal gum of lower incisors, lower canines and pre-molars, and lower lip and chin.

Keyword: Anatomy

Mental nerve block injection
This method of administering local anaesthetic will numb the nerve supplying sensation to all the lower teeth, their buccal or labial gingiva including half the side of the tongue and lip. The most common is the inferior dental block.

Keyword: Anatomy

Mercury (Hg)
A chemical element that is liquid at room temperature. In dentistry, this metal is present in very small quantities in amalgam fillings.

Keyword: Restoration

Mercury poisoning
Mercury vapours are toxic if inhaled or ingested. Its toxic effect can cause symptoms such as headache, nausea and diarrhoea and can progress to severe hand tremors, numbness and visual impairment. If deposits are present in the kidneys, this could lead to kidney failure.

Keyword: Fillings/health and safety

Mershon band pusher
This chisel-like instrument is used during orthodontic procedures to assist in the seating of a band to a tooth.

Keyword: Orthodontic

Mesial tooth surface
This is the surface of the tooth closest to the mid-line facing the front of the tooth.

Keyword: Anatomy

M

Mesioangular impaction
This describes a tooth that is tilted forwards, mesially into the distal aspect of the second molar.

Keyword: Anatomy

Messing gun
A specialised amalgam carrier allowing very small amounts of amalgam to be deposited during the placement of a retrograde filling during an apicectomy.

Keyword: Surgical endodontic

Metal retainer wings
These are fused on either side of the pontic of an adhesive bridge to provide retention. The wings are bonded to the back of the retaining teeth.

Keyword: Prosthetic

Metal ruler
Can be sterilised in the autoclave, and comes in various lengths and used to measure the length of files during a root canal procedure.

Keyword: Endodontic

Metronidazole
An antibiotic drug used to treat infection in dentistry such as ANUG and periocoronitis. It is given to patients who are allergic to penicillin.

Keyword: Drugs

Miconazole
An anti-fungal drug used to treat soreness of the mouth, denture stomatitis, inflammation and dry lips. It can be applied topically as a cream or given orally as a pastille.

Keyword: Drugs

Microbes
The name given to a group of particularly harmful micro-organisms that cause disease, such as fungi, bacteria and viruses.

Keyword: Microbiology

M

Microdontia
These are abnormally small teeth erupting in normal sized jaws.
This type of malocclusion will result in spacing in the jaws.

Keyword: Orthodontic

Micro-organisms
A single-celled living organism of microscopic size. Most are
harmless but some of these germs can play a part in dental
disease, decay and gum disease.

Keyword: Microbiology

Midazolam
A drug used in the emergency treatment of epilepsy, it can also
be administered intravenously to produce sedation, causing
drowsiness and amnesia.

Keyword: Drugs

Middle superior dental nerve
A branch of the maxillary division of the trigeminal nerve. The
nerve supplies the pre-molar teeth and the mesial half of the
molars and their buccal gingiva.

Keyword: Anatomy

Miller forceps
These secure articulating paper in place whilst the patient bites
up and down on it to check their occlusion or any high spots on
restorations.

Keyword: Restorations

Minerals
These are essential to our diet and vital for health. The main
sources of minerals are calcium, phosphates and iron. Minerals,
like vitamins, are introduced to the body in small amounts in
certain food groups or trace elements. They are responsible for
cell structure and function.

Keyword: Digestion

M

Minnesota retractor

Used mainly during surgical procedures providing a clear field of vision for the operator by retracting the cheek and tongue and protects the soft tissue.

Keyword: Minor oral surgery

Mitchell's trimmer

Looks like a carver, cord packer or large excavator. Used during surgical procedures to raise a gum flap or to remove soft tissue for a biopsy.

Keyword: Minor oral surgery

Mitral valve

Situated in the left side of the heart allowing one way blood flow from the left atrium into the left ventricle.

Keyword: Heart and circulation

Mixed dentition

Deciduous and adult teeth are both present in a patient between the ages of six and twelve.

Keyword: Anatomy

Modelling wax

Used during the process of making prosthetic teeth at certain stages. It is used to record jaw relationship and can be softened with warm water or heat.

Keyword: Prosthetic

Modules

Used during orthodontic treatment to hold archwire in place. Held by ligature pliers the module is placed around the bracket. They come in a wide range of colours and materials.

Keyword: Orthodontic

Molar

There are two deciduous molars, D and E, two either side in the mandible and two either side in the maxilla. There are three permanent molars 6, 7 and 8; three either side in the mandible and three either side in the maxilla for grinding and chewing food. Upper molars have three roots and lowers have two.

Keyword: Anatomy

M

Mortonson-Cevedent plugger

A restorative instrument used to condense amalgam into its cavity. The working ends are flat and come in various shapes and sizes depending on the size of the cavity.

Keyword: Restorative

Mouth mirror

Enables direct vision of the tooth and is magnified slightly. It can also be used to retract and protect soft tissues.

Keyword: Instruments

Mouth pack

This is a pad of gauze placed over a bleeding socket after a tooth extraction. The patient bites on the pack for a few minutes until the bleeding has stopped and a clot has formed.

Keyword: Extraction/minor oral surgery

Mouth spreader/gag

Used to keep the mouth propped open if the patient is struggling to do so or if they are sedated. Its locking mechanism allows the operator to choose how wide to keep the patient's mouth open.

Keyword: Sedation

Mucocele

A cyst or swollen mucus-filled sac which can occur when a salivary gland is blocked. They normally appear on the inside of the lower lip but can be present on the floor and roof of the mouth as well.

Keyword: Oral Examination

Mucus

A thick fluid secreted by mucous membranes in order to lubricate and protect parts of the body lined with the membranes.

Keyword: Anatomy

Mucous membrane

This skin-like layer lines the floor of the mouth covering the cheeks, palate and tongue. It contains millions of cells in fluid that is secreted to lubricate and cleanse. The buccal sulcus is the

M

membrane lining the cheeks, and the labial sulcus is the membrane between the lips and teeth.

Keyword: Anatomy

Mucoperiosteum
A mucous membrane attached to the periosteum, covering the bone surface.

Keyword: Anatomy

Mylohyoid line
This ridge marks the floor of the mouth in the inner surface of the body of the mandible.

Keyword: Anatomy

Myocardial infarction
A blockage in the blood supply to the heart causing sudden death to part of the heart muscle. This is also known as a heart attack. Symptoms are severe pain, pale and clammy, low blood pressure and breathing disorders.

Keyword: Collapse

M

N

Nabers probe
Used during a dental examination to detect calculus, caries, margins of restorations, crowns and bridges. Can be single or double ended and the working ends may be straight or curved.

Keyword: Examination

Nance pliers
Used during orthodontic procedures to bend archwires, the beaks that grasp the archwire will vary with the type of archwire used.

Keyword: Orthodontic

National Health Service (NHS)
The public healthcare system in the United Kingdom.

Keyword: Service

NVQ assessor
An individual who holds a certification recognised by the GDC for registration, and has been awarded the A1 qualification. An assessor must have occupational competence, expertise and experience. Their role is to observe trainees working towards NVQ qualification in their workplace, determining the competence of the trainee as well as providing help, support and advice. They will also grade all evidence that is submitted by trainees in their portfolio, awarding criteria related to the standards provided by City & Guilds.

Keyword: Training

Necrosis
This is the death of cells and tissues resulting in inadequate blood supply. Necrosis of the pulp can occur when a tooth becomes non-vital.

Keyword: Endodontic

Needle
Various types and lengths are available depending on the area of the mouth that is being treated. The shorter end of the needle is unsheathed and will puncture the rubber diaphragm of the local anaesthetic cartridge once inside the syringe.

Keyword: Local anaesthetic

Needle stick injury
See Inoculation injury

Needle stick protector
Many different types are available. The needle cap is removed to expose the needle and the cap is placed into a protective sheath. This enables the needle to be placed back into the cap after use safely and securely, avoiding injury.

Keyword: Local anaesthetic

Nervous system
This consists of the brain, spinal cord, nerves and sensory organs. Information is gathered and stored here and controls the body through automatic responses to stimuli. The two divisions of the nervous system are automatic and somatic. The automatic is concerned with unconscious regulation of internal body functions and somatic controls the muscles responsible for voluntary movement.

Keyword: Anatomy

NiTi rotary instruments
NiTi stands for nickel titanium. These rotary flexible files are used during root canal treatment to clean and shape the canals. They are available in different lengths and are placed in the endodontic handpiece.

Keyword: Endodontic

N

Nitrous oxide (N_2O)

A gas that is used in dentistry during inhalation sedation in conjunction with oxygen (O_2). It is a powerful analgesic gas used with special equipment by trained staff.

Keyword: Sedation

Non-milk extrinsic sugars (NMES)

These added sugars in food can increase the risk of tooth decay. This additive is added to foods during the processing stage, NMES are added to biscuits, soft drinks and breakfast cereal and are directly responsible for the start of the tooth decay process.

Keyword: Digestion/oral health disease

Non-pathogenic

Micro-organisms that do not cause disease.

Keyword: Cross-infection control

Non-vital

This term refers to a tooth with a non-vital/dead pulp that is not receiving any blood supply. The pulp has been removed from the inner structure of the tooth by endodontic treatment because it presented with signs of it dying or because the tooth was necrotic.

Keyword: Endodontic

Nylon band seater

Whilst seating an orthodontic band, the patient will be instructed to bite down on this instrument to enable the band to be fixed into position.

Keyword: Orthodontic

Nystatin

An antifungal drug which is used to treat candida albicans (thrush). Can be taken as pastilles.

Keyword: Drugs

O

Obturator
This appliance is made from elastic, acrylic, gutta percha, impression material or soft lining material. It is a permanent appliance used for the plugging of an abnormal cavity, for example a cleft palate or surgical removal of part of the jaw. A denture can have the plug fitted to it to seal this type of cavity.

Keyword: Prosthetic

Occlusal radiograph
A type of intra-oral x-ray providing an image of the maxillary and mandibular arch. Used mainly to check the eruption of teeth.

Keyword: Orthodontic

Occlusal registration
Done using various materials or pastes to record the bite between the tooth being prepared for prosthesis and those which will bite against it.

Keyword: Prosthetic

Occlusal rests
These tiny protrusions are added to a partial denture supporting any metal framework by slotting onto the occlusal surface of the enamel of the remaining natural tooth or a groove cut into a filling.

Keyword: Prosthetics

Occlusal tooth surface
This is the biting surface of all the pre-molars and molars.

Keyword: Anatomy

Occlusion
This describes the relationship between the upper and lower teeth when the jaw is shut.

Keyword: Anatomy

Occlusion rims
Laboratory made and used during the wax-bite stage of denture construction. The rims are worn by the patient and the bite registration is recorded measuring the distance between the upper and lower jaw in its relaxed state.

Keyword: Prosthetic

Ochsenbein chisel
A surgical instrument to remove and smooth bone.

Keyword: Minor oral surgery

Odontoblasts
Connective tissue cells that form the dentine under the tooth enamel and carry on doing so throughout life. These cells are contained in the outer surface of the dental pulp.

Keyword: Anatomy

Oesophagus
This muscular tube is part of the digestive tract; it carries food to the pharynx then to the stomach. The mucous membrane that lines the oesophagus acts with the muscle performing a peristaltic action to move swallowed food down the stomach.

Keyword: Digestion

Omega pliers
An orthodontic instrument. Its grooved beaks are used to bend archwire into loops.

Keyword: Orthodontic

Opaque film
An x-ray that has been over-developed or over-exposed can appear black and opaque. This can be seen by holding the developed film up to the light. Manual developing can cause problems if the developer solution is not at the correct temperature or dilu-

tion. A thermometer will help determine correct processing time.

Keyword: Radiography

Open drainage
Allowing infected pus to drain out of a tooth that has been opened in order to gain access to the necrotic pulp during endodontic treatment.

Keyword: Endodontic

Operculectomy
This is the surgical removal of the gingival flap (operculum) which is present over an erupting wisdom tooth. The flap can be bitten on causing pain and inflammation which could lead to infection.

Keyword: Minor oral surgery

Operculum
This flap of mucosa lies most commonly over partially erupted wisdom teeth.

Keyword: Anatomy

Opposing arch
This refers to the arch which is not receiving the treatment to have a fixed prosthetic. An impression is taken of the opposing arch to determine the correct occlusion when constructing the prosthesis.

Keyword: Prosthetic

Oral cancer
Cancer which can affect anywhere in the oral cavity including soft tissues, salivary glands and bones. If signs are detected early then chances of survival are improved. Signs to look for are ulcers and lumps which have been present for more than 3–6 weeks, white or red patches that may be sore, persistent numbness in the throat and swelling of the neck and jaw.

Keyword: Oral disease

Oral disease
Gingivitis, periodontitis and caries are diseases of the teeth and gums. Poor oral hygiene and poor diet are contributing factors to oral disease.

Keyword: Oral disease

Oral hygiene
This includes many preventive measures to keep the mouth, teeth and gums healthy and reduce the risk of tooth decay and other oral diseases. These measures include tooth brushing, interdental cleaning, oral hygiene instruction, toothbrush instruction and regular check ups and visits to the hygienist.

Keyword: Prevention

Oral sedation
Also called premedication. A tranquilliser is given to a patient to take orally before treatment to relieve anxiety. Diazepam is usually prescribed to be taken the night before and temazepam is taken one hour before treatment.

Keyword: Drugs

Orange ring conventional handpiece
It has variable speeds and runs faster than the speed of the motor. Latch grip attachments are used with it.

Keyword: Handpieces and burs

Orbicularis oculi
A ring of muscle that surrounds each eye connecting with muscles to produce movements of facial expression.

Keyword: Anatomy

Orbicularis oris
A ring of muscle that surrounds the mouth producing movements of facial expression.

Keyword: Anatomy

Oro-antral fistula
This means an opening between the oral cavity and maxillary sinus caused by a perforation made during an extraction of an upper pre-molar or molar close to the floor of the maxillary sinus.

If the perforation is large, there will be air bubbles in the socket or fluid will enter the nose after drinking. This will need to be closed.

Keyword: Extraction/minor oral surgery

Oropharyngeal airway
See Guedel airway

Ortho band
Used during orthodontic procedures. They are cemented on to posterior teeth and archwires are secured by its hooked tube.

Keyword: Orthodontic

Ortho bracket
Used during the fitting of an orthodontic appliance and cemented to the buccal surface of the tooth to help secure archwires.

Keyword: Orthodontic

Ortho bracket card
Orthodontic brackets stick to this card and keep them in the correct order of placement in the mouth. This system enables placement to be done quickly.

Keyword: Orthodontic

Orthodontics
Ortho means correct, normal or straight. This branch of dentistry concentrates on a patient's malocclusion and how to treat this by designing and providing a removable or fixed appliance to treat the patient's specific needs.

Keyword: Orthodontics

Orthopantomograph (OPG)
This extra-oral x-ray image will show all of the teeth and supporting structures including sinuses, bone, joints, nerves, roots, impacted and unerupted teeth.

Keyword: Radiography

Osteoclast cell
A large cell involved in the modelling and formation of the bone. It is responsible for the absorption of bone when it is being restructured under stress, such as orthodontic treatment. The

cells eat the bone enabling movement of the tooth root in this direction.

Keyword: Anatomy

Osteotome kit

This is a set of instruments used in implant placement to prepare the bone. They are either straight or angled for access to the posterior maxilla and are used primarily in the maxilla or where bone quality is poor to try and increase the density of the osteotomy.

Keyword: Implants

Overbite

This shows how much the upper incisors slightly overlap the lowers vertically, tilting backwards slightly. If the overbite is greater than 50% then it is a class II division 1 bite and an orthodontic referral may be needed to correct this.

Keyword: Orthodontics

Over denture

Can be made as a full or partial denture that fits on standing teeth or retained roots. The roots remaining are not extracted so as not to cause shrinkage of the alveolar bone. This mostly occurs with lower dentures which have the most problem with bone shrinkage and loose fitting dentures.

Keyword: Prosthetic

Overjet

This shows how much the upper incisors slightly overlap the lowers, horizontally. If the measurement records more than a 2–4 mm overjet, this is a class II division 1 bite.

Keyword: Orthodontics

Oxygen (O$_2$)

An essential gas that is absorbed through the lungs, into the blood circulating around the body and into the tissues. Oxygen is necessary for turning food into energy through metabolism.

Keyword: Physiology

Palatal connecting bar

This is incorporated to a spring cantilever bridge connecting the pontic to the retainer when they are several teeth away from each other.

Keyword: Prosthetic

Palatal finger spring

This type of spring is added to a removable orthodontic appliance to retract the canine and pre-molar teeth.

Keyword: Orthodontic

Palatal tooth surface

This is the surface of all upper teeth closer to the roof of the mouth.

Keyword: Anatomy

Palate

The roof of the mouth separating the mouth from the nasal cavity. It is covered with a mucous membrane. The front is hard and the back is soft. The hard palate forms part of the maxilla, and the soft protects the pharynx.

Keyword: Anatomy

Pancreas

This gland lies beneath the stomach and the abdomen. It secretes digestive enzymes into the duodenum along with sodium bicarbonate to neutralise stomach acid. Its hormone function secretes insulin and glycogen to regulate the level of glucose in the blood.

Keyword: Anatomy

Panoramic radiograph
See Orthopantomograph (OPG)

Paper points
Used during endodontic procedures. Placed in the root canal to absorb any moisture such as blood, pus and saliva. Also used to place medicaments into the canal.

Keyword: Endodontic

Paracetamol
An analgesic drug mainly used to treat mild pain such as head-ache, it also reduces fever.

Keyword: Drugs

Paraesthesia
An altered sensation in the skin caused by the effect of local anaesthetic wearing off. A tingling sensation like pins and needles will occur.

Keyword: Local anaesthetic

Parallax
This radiographic technique is the change of the angular position of an object being exposed to x-rays.

Keyword: Radiography

Paralleling technique
A radiographic technique which involves the x-ray machine being held parallel to the long axis of the tooth being exposed. This will produce an image that is exactly the same size as the tooth.

Keyword: Radiography

Parotid salivary gland
Largest of three pairs of salivary glands. It is located above the angle of the jaw, and below and in front of the ear on each side of the face. It is connected to the oral cavity via a duct (Stenson's) which opens against the upper molar teeth. Mumps usually affects this gland.

Keyword: Anatomy

Partial denture

Can be made from acrylic or with a metal framework. This type of denture replaces only a few missing teeth on the upper or lower arch.

Keyword: Prosthetic

Partly blank film

An x-ray film that has been exposed can appear as partly blank after processing, this is caused by operator error, such as angulation of the collimator tube. This can also occur during manual processing if films are not fully immersed in the developer tank.

Keyword: Radiation

Pathogen

This is a micro-organism that causes disease; it is also referred to as a germ. An example of a pathogenic infectious disease is tuberculosis. Food and water can also become contaminated with pathogens but food safety regulations and water treatments have reduced the threat of this.

Keyword: Cross-infection control

Patient relief wax

Bees' wax that is used on a fixed orthodontic appliance to relieve trauma to the soft tissues. The wax will cover the part of the appliance causing the trauma and protects the soft tissue until healing; the appliance will need adjusting.

Keyword: Orthodontic

Penicillin

An antibiotic drug used to treat infective conditions.

Keyword: Drugs

Performance criteria

This relates to the NVQ standards set out by City & Guilds. The performance of a trainee in the workplace will be observed by an NVQ assessor or expert witness. There are performance criteria in the standards that must be met in order to achieve the qualification.

Keyword: Training

Periapical periodontitis
Inflammation of the tissues surrounding the teeth causing toothache when biting. A cyst may occur causing swelling in the jaw.

Keyword: Periodontal Disease

Periapical radiograph
An intra-oral x-ray; the image will show the entire tooth of interest including the root and supporting structures. Usually taken to diagnose an abscess, cyst or decay under a filling. The length of a root is a diagnostic for measuring the file from the apex during endodontic treatment.

Keyword: Radiography

Periocoronitis
This is the inflammation of the gum overlying the erupting tooth, usually a partially erupted third molar. It can occur on any tooth but normally resolves when the tooth is fully erupted. When involving the wisdom teeth, further problems can occur leading to infection.

Keyword: Periodontal disease

Periodontal disease
A disorder of the tissues that surround and support the teeth. Periodontitis is the inflammation of these tissues.

Keyword: Periodontal disease

Periodontal ligament
This fibrous tissue that holds the tooth in place between the tooth and tooth socket. It acts as a shock absorber resisting the stresses of chewing. It contains blood vessels and sensory nerve endings making them sensitive to excessive pressure.

Keyword: Anatomy

Periodontal probe
Measures the depth of the periodontal pockets around the gingival crevice. The measurements are recorded in millimetres using this blunt probe so as not to cause trauma. The measurements will indicate if there is any bone loss, gingival recession and detects sub-gingival calculus.

Keyword: Periodontal disease

Periodontics
This is the branch of dentistry concerned with prevention, diagnosis and treatment of periodontal disease, this relates to tissues that surround and support the teeth.

Keyword: Periodontal disease

Periosteal elevator
Used during surgical procedures for retraction purposes, this instrument holds the tissue from the bone enabling a clear field of vision to the site.

Keyword: Minor oral surgery

P

Periotome
Used during surgical extraction procedures to elevate the tooth and roots from the socket causing less trauma and damage to the bone in case an implant can be placed later. Periotomes are double ended with a curved and a straight edge. One end is used for posterior teeth and the other for anterior.

Keyword: Extractions/minor oral surgery

Peristalsis
The movement of food and waste products through the digestive system. The wave-like movement is caused by the muscular contraction and relaxation of the smooth muscles in the walls of the digestive tract and ureters.

Keyword: Digestion

Personal protective equipment (PPE)
This includes masks, safety glasses, gloves, visors, aprons, bibs, gowns, hats and other parts of the uniform provided to staff or patients to help in the prevention of cross-infection and to promote health and safety.

Keyword: Health and safety/Cross-infection control

Peeso reamer drill
An endodontic instrument that attaches into a conventional handpiece and is used to remove gutta percha (rubber) from the canal during the preparation of a post. They come in various sizes and clear the way for a suitable length post to be placed to

provide retention for a crown when most of the natural tooth is lost.

Keyword: Endodontic/restorative

pH

This is the measurement of the acidity or alkalinity of a solution. The scale ranges from 0–14, 7 being neutral. The pH of the body is close to 7.4, as is the oral cavity. Acid conditions range from 0–7 and alkaline conditions range from 8–14. if the pH drops to 5.5, this acid condition will cause tooth demineralisation. Minerals contained in saliva will take two hours to neutralise the acid and return to pH7.

Keyword: Oral disease

Pharynx

A cone-shaped passage connecting the back of the mouth and nose to the oesophagus. The upper part is the nasopharynx, the middle part is the oropharynx and the lower part is called the laryngopharynx. It forms the open cavity of the throat from nose to mouth and enables the swallowing mechanism to function.

Keyword: Digestion

Plaque

This is responsible for the main part of tooth decay and gingivitis. The sticky coating consists of saliva, bacteria and food debris. Some of the micro-organisms in plaque create an acid that eats away at tooth enamel.

Keyword: Caries

Plasma

The liquid portion of the blood in which you find blood cells. It is mostly water and contains plasma proteins. It carries nutrients to the cells of various organs in the body and transports waste products to the kidneys, liver and lungs for excretion. It contains antibodies and antitoxins to give resistance to disease. Plasma also plays a part in the blood clotting process.

Keyword: Blood

Plaster

A material used to cast models from impressions taken with alginate. Various types are available.

Keyword: Impressions

Plastic instrument

Used to deliver filling material to the cavity without sticking or discolouring it.

Keyword: Restorative

Platelets

The smallest type of blood cells, also called thrombocytes. Their primary functions are to stop bleeding by clotting or coagulation.

Keyword: Blood

Pocket mask

Part of an emergency kit. This mask contains a one-way valve to prevent fluids passing between first aider and victim. The mask is placed over the individual's mouth and the first aider breathes into the mouthpiece.

Keyword: Emergency Procedure/First Aid

Polishing/finishing strips

Long, abrasive strips used to polish composite fillings interproximally. The strips have varying degrees of abrasiveness and can also be used to remove interproximal staining.

Keyword: Restorative

Polycarboxylate cement

A powder and liquid mixed together and used as cement for fixing crowns, it can also be used as a lining. It consists of zinc oxide and polyacrylic acid

Keyword: Restorative

Polyether

Very accurate impression materials used for prosthetic work. The two pastes are mixed together in equal quantities and loaded into a special syringe and placed on the prepared tooth. The remainder of the material is placed in an impression tray and a mould taken of the tooth.

Keyword: Impressions

Porcelain
A material that veneers and crowns are made of and can be used to make part of a prosthetic. It is delicate and can fracture under a heavy bite.

Keyword: Restorative/prosthetic

Portal vein
This large vein carries digested food from the stomach to the liver.

Keyword: Digestion

Post crown
This type of crown is cemented onto a metal post and core which is inserted into an empty root canal of a non-vital tooth providing a permanent restoration.

Keyword: Restorative

Posterior band remover
Used to remove posterior orthodontic bands, the tip of the instrument is placed on the occlusal surface and the beak placed at the gingival edge.

Keyword: Orthodontic

Posterior superior dental nerve
One of the five branches of the maxillary division. Its nerve supplies the distal half of the 1st, 2nd and 3rd molar teeth including their buccal gingivae.

Keyword: Anatomy

Prefabricated post kit
Contains drills and posts of varying sizes. The correct size is placed in the root of the tooth providing retention and a superstructure (the crown) is placed on top of the tooth.

Keyword: Restorative

Premedication

These are drugs, such as a tranquillisers, given before surgery to help with anxiety.

Keyword: Drugs

Pre-molar

Two in the upper and two in the lower jaw located on each side of the mouth between the canines and molar teeth. They have two roots: buccal or palatal in the upper jaw, and buccal or lingual in the lower jaw.

Keyword: Anatomy

Prescriptions

A written instruction of a particular drug written by a dentist or doctor directing a pharmacist on what medication has been prescribed to the patient. The pharmacist will then give the patient the prescribed medication.

Keyword: Drugs

Pressure relief paste

This paste is placed on a denture that is causing discomfort and will detect high spots on the affected surface so that the denture can be eased.

Keyword: Prosthetic

Pressure systems

Autoclaves and air receivers with a capacity of more than 250 bar litres must comply with the Pressure Systems Safety Regulations 2000. Serious injury can occur from the release of stored energy as a result of a pressure systems failure, such as explosive displacement of the door, violent opening of the door immediately after a completed cycle and explosion of sealed gases. Therefore, training should be given to all persons using such equipment. This is enforced under the Provision and Use of Work Equipment Regulations 1998. All autoclaves have a safety valve to prevent over-pressurisation. The maximum allowable working pressure is marked and autoclaves with quick opening doors do not pressurise unless door is completely closed.

Keyword: Health and safety

Pre-sterilisation cleaning

This is the first stage of the decontamination process. Contaminated instruments that have been in contact with oral and body fluids, such as blood and saliva, must be cleaned before sterilisation by autoclave. This can be done by hand scrubbing them, although the preferred methods are ultrasonic cleaning or using a washer disinfector. Hand scrubbing instruments can cause inoculation injuries if not done carefully and is not as effective.

Keyword: Cross-infection control

Prilocaine

A generic name for Citanest®. A local anaesthetic drug that does not contain adrenaline; used for patients who have heart conditions or blood-pressure related problems. The numbing sensation of this anaesthetic does not last for long, therefore it is used for treatment that does not take very long to do.

Keyword: Drugs

Primary haemorrhage

This occurs within the first five minutes of a tooth being extracted and is caused by blood vessels being torn in the periodontium. It is normal and bleeding will stop once a clot has formed.

Keyword: Extraction/Minor Oral Surgery

Prion (from proteinaceous infectious virion)

A prion is a tiny protein-based infectious particle that can transmit diseases such as CJD. The prion protein cannot be destroyed by normal methods of sterilisation and no treatment is available for prion diseases.

Keyword: Pathology

Probe

Used during a basic periodontal examination (BPE). Its blunt ball working end measures the depth of the periodontal pockets and detects sub-gingival calculus. The probe has bands on it measured in millimetres and the six sextants of the arches are measured only with this probe.

Keyword: Periodontal

Professional complementary to dentistry (PCD)
The name given to all members of the dental team other than dentists.

Keyword: Governing body

Prophy angle attachment
These are disposable and attach to a conventional handpiece. A polishing cup or brush are fitted and used to polish teeth. The single use is designed to reduce cross-infection.

Keyword: Periodontal

Prophy conventional handpiece
Disposable polishing cups or brushes used to polish teeth screw on to this handpiece and are then placed on a motor running at 40,000 rpm.

Keyword: Periodontal

Prophylaxis
Meaning the prevention of disease. Preventive measures designed to prevent the occurrence of disease such as antibiotic cover. Sometimes abbreviated as prophy.

Keyword: Drugs

Prophy ring
A single dose of prophylaxis paste is held securely by this ring and placed on the operator's finger.

Keyword: Periodontal

Propofol
An intravenous anaesthetic drug which produces immediate unconsciousness.

Keyword: Drugs

Prosthetic
These replace missing teeth and include supporting structures such as dentures, bridges and implants. There are fixed and removable prosthetic appliances.

Keyword: Prosthetic

Protein

Proteins are broken down in the stomach into amino acids during digestion. Protein is necessary for maintaining tissues and for cell growth and repair. Dietary sources of protein include meat, fish, eggs, milk and cheese.

Keyword: Digestion

P

Ptyalin

An enzyme also called a salivary amylase. It is responsible for the digestive action of saliva, initiating the digestive action of carbohydrates.

Keyword: Digestion

Pulmonary artery

Pulmonary means anything relating to the lungs. This artery carries oxygen-depleted blood to the lungs for oxygenation and removal of excess carbon dioxide. The blood passes out of the right ventricle through the pulmonary artery to the lungs.

Keyword: Heart and circulation

Pulmonary vein

Transports oxygenated blood from the lungs to the left upper chamber of the heart.

Keyword: Heart and circulation

Pulp

Located in the middle of each tooth. It is a soft tissue containing blood vessels and sensory nerves allowing the tooth to feel hot, cold, touch and pain. The tissue is contained in the pulp chamber.

Keyword: Anatomy

Pulp capping

An endodontic procedure which involves placing a calcium hydroxide dressing over the exposed vital pulp and covered with a matrix cap and sedative zinc oxide cement until it can be restored. Reparative dentine formation will occur allowing the tooth to repair the exposure site. If this fails then root canal treatment is required.

Keyword: Endodontic

Pulpectomy

This endodontic procedure is involved in the removal of the tooth pulp.

Keyword: Endodontic

Pulpitis

The main cause of this is pulp exposure and can lead to the death of the pulp. If the pulp has become infected by bacteria entering the exposed pulp, root canal treatment or extraction is required.

Keyword: Endodontic

Pulpotomy

The procedure involves the removal of the coronal part of the tooth after it has become inflamed by infection.

Keyword: Endodontic

Pulse

The dilation of an artery as blood is forced through it pumped by the heart. The rhythmic pulse can be felt by applying fingertip pressure to the skin where arteries travel near its surface, for example the carotid artery of the neck.

Keyword: Heart and circulation

Pulse oximeter

A portable device enabling the reading of the pulse rate of a patient. Required when IV sedation is carried out.

Keyword: Sedation

Pus

A fluid found at the site of bacterial infections. Contains millions of dead white blood cells, digested tissue and bacteria. A collection of pus is also called an abscess.

Keyword: Infection

Push scaler

Used during periodontal procedures to remove supra-gingival calculus and plaque. Can be single or double ended to use on anterior or posterior teeth.

Keyword: Periodontal

Q

Quality Assurance (QA)

Quality assurance in dental radiography ensures that practices are keeping radiation doses to patients as low as reasonably practicable by achieving high standards of image quality, good diagnostic quality, maintenance of equipment, correct methods of film processing and adequate training. A number of radiographs should be viewed, rated and analysed. Radiographs that present with poor quality should be further assessed to identify causes and if improvements need to be made in operator techniques or developing methods.

Keyword: Radiography

R

Radiation
Emissions of energy in the form of electromagnetic waves or particles from unstable atoms. Radiation can be harmful in large doses but is useful in diagnosis and treatments.

Keyword: Radiography

Radiation monitoring badge
See Dosimeter

Radiation protection advisor (RPA)
An RPA advises a dental practice on how to comply with all relevant regulations relating to x-rays and equipment. The RPA is a medical/physics expert trained in all aspects of radiation protection.

Keyword: Radiography

Radiation protection file
This file should be kept in the practice and contains information such as local rules, working instructions, contingency plans, dose investigation level and written procedures for patient protection. Staff training and courses attended can also be included. This file needs to be revised regularly and kept up-to-date.

Keyword: Radiography

Radiation protection supervisor (RPS)
This trained person in the dental practice will hold a certificate in Dental Radiography. The RPS will supervise all aspects of radiography in the practice.

Keyword: Radiography

Radicular pulp

This is the part of the pulp contained within the apical/root portion of the tooth.

Keyword: Endodontic

Radiography

This is the use of radiation, such as x-rays, to provide images of the teeth, jaws, soft tissues, sinuses, etc.

Keyword: Radiography

Radiolucent

Relating to anything that permits the penetration of x-rays when exposed. This substance will appear dark on the developed x-ray.

Keyword: Radiography

Radiopaque

Relating to anything that blocks the penetration of x-rays when exposed. The image will appear lighter on a developed x-ray.

Keyword: Radiography

Rake retractor

Used during surgical procedures to retract the mucoperiosteal flap (composed of mucosa and periosteum), protecting the tissues and gingiva and giving a clear field of vision.

Keyword: Minor oral surgery

Ratchet wrench

Part of a dental implant kit used to seat the implant.

Keyword: Implants

Reactionary haemorrhage

This is bleeding several hours after an extraction because the clot has been disturbed. Pressure is applied to the socket again until bleeding stops.

Keyword: Extractions/minor oral surgery

Reamer

An instrument used during endodontic procedures to enlarge a root canal in preparation for the insertion of a root filling. The instruments come in increasing widths to enable the canal to be widened. They are colour coded by size and can be used as hand instruments or attached to a handpiece.

Keyword: Endodontics

Records
These are confidential, detailed and updated files of patients and should be stored in a locked cabinet, cupboard or on a computer. The records include medical history, treatment plans, correspondence, payments, x-rays and other patient information. Patient notes should be as detailed as possible and should only be viewed by those who have the right to do so.

Keyword: Administration/confidentiality

Rectum
Located at the end of the large intestine and connected to the anus. This short muscular tube carries waste to the anus to be eliminated from the body.

Keyword: Anatomy

Red blood cells
These cells float in blood plasma and carry oxygen to the body cells. They contain haemoglobin, enzymes, minerals and sugars. Haemoglobin is a pigment that gives the cells their red colour.

Keyword: Anatomy

Red ribbon wax
Used during the bite and try-in stages of denture construction as well as for crowns and bridges. It can be added to impression trays to extend the height and length.

Keyword: Restorations/prosthetics

Relative anaesthesia (RA)
Also known as inhalation sedation. A mixture of nitrous oxide (N_2O) and oxygen (O_2) form an analgesic gas supplied in cylinders. The gas is administered through a nose mask whilst a qualified operator controls the machine. To prevent overdose, the maximum N_2O level is 50% and O_2 is 30%.

Keyword: Sedation

Remineralisation
This is the action of the enamel being restored and repaired by fluoride after the areas of the enamel have been attacked by acid causing demineralisation.

Keyword: Caries

Removable orthodontic appliance
Worn by an individual who is undergoing orthodontic treatment. Its base is acrylic and has a stainless steel component holding the appliance to the teeth. The appliance can easily be removed for cleaning.

Keyword: Orthodontic

Removable prosthetic appliances
This refers to any laboratory-made appliances that can be removed from the oral cavity such as dentures, removable braces, mouth guards and shields.

Keyword: Prosthetics

Resorption
This is the loss of substance from teeth such as dentine, alveolar bone and cementum. Primary teeth are lost by this process. Resorption of the roots means that the teeth become loose. After an extraction osteoclast cells eat away at the alveolar bone reducing the alveolar ridge.

Keyword: Anatomy

Respiration
This is breathing. Oxygen(O_2) enters the blood and carbon dioxide (CO_2) leaves. Air containing oxygen is breathed into the lungs through the alveoli and diffuses into the blood carrying it to the cells in the body. Carbon dioxide is produced as a waste product and passes into the blood from the body cells where it is transported to the lungs and breathed out.

Keyword: Anatomy/breathing

Respiratory system
This includes all of the organs responsible for carrying oxygen from the air to the blood and expelling carbon dioxide.

Keyword: Anatomy

Resuscitation
See Basic life support

Retroclined
This describes the angulations of the upper central incisor teeth when they appear to be sloping backwards into the mouth.

Keyword: Orthodontic

Retrograde root filling
This is an amalgam filling placed in the bone cavity where the apex of the root has been amputated during an apicectomy. A special fine-bore amalgam carrier is used to deliver small amounts of filling into the cavity.

Keyword: Surgical endodontics

Reversible pulpitis
If the inflamed pulp has been treated by removing the caries then endodontic treatment is not necessary and the tooth can be permanently restored. The tooth will heal itself over time.

Keyword: Endodontic

Reye's Syndrome
It is very important to know that if aspirin is prescribed to children under the age of 16, it may cause a rare but fatal brain disorder. Studies show that aspirin is a predisposing factor in developing this condition. Symptoms are vomiting, memory loss, lethargy, seizures and breathing problems.

Keyword: Drugs/disease

Rheumatic fever
A rare condition, especially in developed countries. Symptoms present as painful and swollen joints, patches and lumps on the skin and heart tissue and valves can become damaged. The exact cause is still unknown but it usually develops after certain strains of the Streptococci bacteria, for example strep throat. If a patient has had rheumatic fever, this needs to be recorded in their medical history as damage could have been caused to the heart valves. Antibiotic cover is needed one hour prior to treatments that may cause the gums to bleed.

Keyword: Pathology

RIDDOR (Reporting of Injuries, Disease and Dangerous Occurrences Regulations)

These incidents must be reported to the Health and Safety Executive as soon as possible and recorded in a special accident book. Guidelines for carrying out these procedures and classifications of what would define a major injury or dangerous occurrence should be kept in the practice's health and safety folder for everyone to read.

Keyword: Health and safety

Right angle probe

Used to feel cavity margins, detect soft dentine and over-hanging restorations.

Keyword: Basic instruments

Risk assessment

Health and safety risks are assessed in the practice, protecting workers and visitors from potential accidents and incidents. Hazards are identified and individuals who might be at risk are identified and precautions and control measures are implemented.

Keyword: Health and safety

Roberts retractor

A type of spring used on a removable orthodontic appliance to reduce a large overjet involving all incisors.

Keyword: Orthodontics

Root canal explorer

Used during endodontic procedures to detect canal openings.

Keyword: Endodontic

Root canal hand file

See Endodontic K file

Rotary paste filler

Sometimes referred to as a spiral filler. Used during endodontic procedures and attaches to a handpiece. Material is added to this flexible instrument and placed into the root canal, rotating the paste for coverage.

Keyword: Endodontic

Rubber cup
Used to polish teeth after a scale has been done, prophylaxis polishing paste is usually added to the cup to remove stains from the tooth surface.

Keyword: Handpieces and attachments

Rubber dam
A thin sheet of rubber that attaches to a frame and is placed over the tooth that the operator is treating, isolating it from other teeth. This provides a clear field of vision for the operator, makes aspirating easier and the patient can still swallow shielding their tongue from the tooth. This helps with moisture control, cross-infection, health and safety and prevents small instruments from being accidentally dropped into the oral cavity. Debris and water from the drilling of the tooth or any filling material will not enter the patient's mouth. It is used during endodontic procedures and fillings.

Keyword: Endodontic/fillings

Rubber dam clamp
Used to remove and place rubber dam clamps around a tooth securing the rubber dam. They are spring loaded and its beaks fit into the holes of the clamp for secure placement.

Keyword: Endodontic

Rubber dam punch
Used to punch holes in to the rubber dam sheet so it will fit over the tooth being treated.

Keyword: Endodontic

Rubber frame
Made from metal or plastic. The rubber dam is stretched over this frame and positioned over the tooth; it covers most of the mouth keeping the nasal passages clear.

Keyword: Endodontic/restorations

Rubella
A viral infection known as German Measles. During the early stages of pregnancy this virus can cause severe birth defects but only in those women who are not immune. A vaccination is given

to women whilst in secondary school to prevent the disease. The virus is spread through airborne droplets or from mother to baby.

Keyword: Diseases

R

S

Safety syringes
Designed to protect user from inoculation injury with a plastic sheath which covers the needle when not in use. They are easy and safe to use and dispose of.

Keyword: Local anaesthetic

Saliva
This alkaline fluid is secreted into the mouth by the salivary glands and mucous membranes lining the mouth. It has several functions, including lubricating the mouth, breaking down carbohydrates and increasing the sense of taste. Saliva's cleansing properties help neutralise acids.

Keyword: Digestion

Saliva ejectors
Come in various shapes and sizes. They fit into the adapter on low volume suction and can remain in the patient's mouth throughout treatment. They can retract and protect soft tissues and reduce the amount of saliva in the oral cavity.

Keyword: Moisture control

Scaling
A periodontal procedure that maintains a patient's oral health. There are varying degrees of scaling depending on the individual's needs. A simple scale is usually done every three to six months. Some patients require more frequent visits and a lengthier appointment. The procedure involves the use of hand instruments or ultrasonic scaling tips designed to remove plaque and calculus.

Keyword: Periodontal

Scalpel

Available as a handle with fitted blade in sterile single use packages or as a separate handle and blade. The blade is very carefully placed on to the handle enabling the operator to make intra-oral incisions. The blade is disposed of in a sharps container and the metal handle can be sterilised.

Keyword: Minor oral surgery

Secondary haemorrhage

This can occur in the socket of a tooth extraction if the blood clot is disturbed and lost early, within the first 24 hours. This could cause infection by bacteria present in the mouth.

Keyword: Extraction/minor oral surgery

Sectional matrix

The matrix provides a proximal wall during class II restorations on posterior teeth. It is single use and available in different sizes depending on the tooth shape.

Keyword: Restorations

Sedation

Used in different ways to reduce anxiety by use of a drug to calm a person. Can be administered intravenously or by inhalation.

Keyword: Sedation

Self-aspirating local anaesthetic syringe

A disposable needle and local anaesthetic cartridge is fitted to this syringe which can be sterilised. This type of syringe prevents the accidental injection of a blood vessel. If blood is seen flowing back into the cartridge, then the needle needs to be removed and repositioned.

Keyword: Local anaesthetic

Self-reflective account

This is a piece of evidence required to be produced by an individual who is receiving training towards certification via the NVQ Oral Health Care: Dental Nursing course. A clinical procedure such as a surgical extraction may be difficult for the NVQ assessor to observe, typically due to the rare occurrence of such a procedure. A trainee can, in this case, provide a reflective account of the procedure by describing in detail the activities they would expect to perform during such a procedure.

Keyword: Training

Semi-lunar valve

The function of this valve is to prevent regurgitation by stopping blood from flowing backwards from the arteries into the heart. Theses valves are present in the aorta and pulmonary artery.

Keyword: Heart and circulation

Separator placing pliers

An orthodontic instrument used for the interproximal placement of elastic separators.

Keyword: Orthodontic

Sevoflurane

Used for the induction of general anaesthesia when mixed with oxygen and nitrous oxide.

Keyword: Sedation

Shade guide

There are many types depending on manufacturer, restoration and prosthetic being done. Each laboratory should supply shade guides to the practice. When doing white fillings, other restorations and prosthetic work, the guide is used to match the colour of the material or prosthetic to the patient's natural teeth. The shade of any work to be constructed by the lab is written on the lab ticket.

Keyword: Restorations/prosthetics

Sharps container

A special waste container used to store any sharp objects that are used in the surgery such as blades, needles and root canal files. When nearly full the container locks and can not be opened. The containers are puncture and leak proof so that they can be stored safely on the premises until collected by a waste company who call on a regular agreed basis.

Keyword: Health and safety

Sharps injury
See inoculation injury

Sharp ridges
The alveolar bone can present as sharp or rough. This can be due to traumatic extractions or if teeth have been lost at different periods of time, causing bone shrinkage and making the ridge uneven. Surgery can be done to smooth the ridge (alveolectomy) providing a more even surface enabling a better and more comfortable fit for dentures.

Keyword: Prosthetics

Shimstock
Very thin articulating foil; placed in Miller forceps to check a patient's occlusion and any high spots present after restoration or prosthetic appliances fitted.

Keyword: Restorations/prosthetics

Sickle/contra-angled probe
Used during a dental examination to detect calculus, defective fissures and margins. Various types available.

Keyword: Basic instruments

Sickle scaler
A hand instrument used during periodontal procedures to remove supra-gingival calculus and plaque. They have a variety of working ends depending which teeth are being treated.

Keyword: Periodontal

Silane coupling agent
A liquid present in kits used for cementing veneers, crowns and bridges allowing the applied dual-cure resin cement to chemically bond, providing good adhesion.

Keyword: Restorations/prosthetics

Silicone wash impression
This type of impression is taken to provide a hard reline to a denture. The elastic material is added to the denture and placed into the patient's mouth. Once it is set, the denture, with the

added material, will be sent to the laboratory so the reline can be made. This technique provides an accurate impression.

Keyword: Prosthetic

Silver point

Used during endodontic procedures as a root filling material. It is not commonly used.

Keyword: Endodontic

Simple extraction

The removal of a tooth without the need to remove soft tissue or raise a gingival flap to remove root or bone. The tooth will usually come out with the use of forceps and instruments used to elevate and loosen the tooth from the periodontal membrane.

Keyword: Extraction

Simulation

This can replace an activity that cannot be observed, for example a trainee might not be given the opportunity to perform a certain procedure in the workplace, but needs to demonstrate the ability to present knowledge and understanding of a specific subject appropriately. This piece of evidence can be used in the trainee's portfolio and awarded criteria to support the NVQ standards.

Keyword: Training

Single use

These items are to be used once only and then disposed of. Such items include anaesthetic needles, impression trays and scalpel blades.

Keyword: Cross-infection control

Sinus

Cavity or recess in the body. There are many sinuses in the bones of the face and surrounding the nose.

Keyword: Anatomy

Sinus augmentation

Also known as a sinus lift. If the bone in the area above the upper posterior teeth is too soft and shallow it is not suitable for an implant placement. This surgical procedure is therefore carried out, using a bone substitute and placing it in the sinus spaces above the upper posterior teeth where the bone will grow allowing the implant to be placed at a later date.

Keyword: Implants

Siqveland matrix retainer
This retainer holds a disposable metal matrix band which provides proximal walls to pre-molar and molar teeth during filling procedures. The band can be sterilised.

Keyword: Restorations

Skin
Outer body tissue covering and protecting internal organs. It provides insulation and regulates the body's temperature.

Keyword: Anatomy

Skull
The skeleton part of the head housing the brain, mandible and maxilla and forms the facial skeleton. The skull sits on the first cervical vertebra.

Keyword: Anatomy

Slow speed handpiece
This contra-angled handpiece is used with a latch grip bur to remove caries during cavity preparation. Polishing brushes can also be attached.

Keyword: Handpieces/burs

Small intestine
About 5–6 metres in length and divided into three sections; this is where most of the digestion process takes place. The digestive tract ends at the anus when digestion is complete.

Keyword: Digestion

Sociable cleanliness
Appears visibly clean to a socially accepted standard.

Keyword: Cross-infection

Sodium hypochlorite
A solution which can be made from household bleach when mixed with water. It is used to irrigate root canals during endodontic procedures to disinfect and remove debris.

Keyword: Drugs/endodontics

Soft lining

This is added to a loose denture which has lost its fit over a period of time due to the bony ridges in the mouth changing or shrinking. The material added to the denture will act as a temporary solution until a new denture is made which fits and moulds better to the tissues. The hard or soft reline can be made chair side in the practice or sent to a laboratory.

Keyword: Prosthetics

Soft palate

At the back of the hard palate is soft tissue that functions to seal off the oral cavity from the nasal cavity during swallowing.

Keyword: Anatomy

Southend clasp

These types of clasps are present on a removable orthodontic appliance to retain it around the incisors.

Keyword: Orthodontics

Spatula

Used for mixing dental materials. Available in a variety of sizes and types depending on the material that needs mixing. Some spatulas are used so they do not stick to the material or discolour it. They can be single or double ended.

Keyword: Basic instruments

Special trays

These secondary impression trays are made by a laboratory following initial impressions of a patient using standard trays. These trays are made specifically for the individual to give a more accurate impression to go towards the wax try-in stage of denture construction.

Keyword: Prosthetics

Special waste

All special waste in the dental surgery needs to be disposed of safely as it is potentially harmful. Following guidelines carefully will ensure correct and safe methods of storage until collected by a hazardous waste company. The waste is disposed of into correctly labelled containers and bags.

Keyword: Health and safety

Spencer Wells
A name given to suture needle holders. (See Needle holders)

Sphygmomanometer
Apparatus used to measure arterial blood pressure. Its inflatable arm cuff is attached by a tube to a pressure recording device. The cuff is fitted on the upper arm and is inflated to prevent blood flow. When deflated and the blood starts flowing, a stethoscope is used in conjunction with this to listen to the blood flow.

Keyword: Heart and circulation

Spirochaetes
An elongated spiral-shaped bacteria which can be present in the mouth and is one of the bacteria associated with acute necrotising ulcerative gingivitis (ANUG).

Keyword: Microbiology

Spoon curette
Used during a surgical procedure. Looks like a large excavator and is used to remove debris and infectious material from the extraction site.

Keyword: Extractions/minor oral surgery

Spoon denture
This denture is constructed to have a spoon-shaped acrylic connector that sits in the palate. This will only work if one anterior tooth is to be placed on a denture. This means that the gingival margins are not covered by acrylic. If the denture loses its fit due to bone resorption then the anterior tooth on the denture will not appear malaligned with the surrounding natural teeth.

Keyword: Prosthetics

Spoon excavator
Used during restorative procedures to remove debris and soft dentine from the cavity site. Available in various shapes.

Keyword: Basic instruments

Spores
Found in bacteria and have a tough protective coating making them highly resistant. Spores found in the mouth are associated with chronic periodontal disease.

Keyword: Periodontal

Stagnation area
Caries are most likely to occur in surfaces of the teeth where food will collect, such as in fissures and interproximal spaces. Bacteria will flourish in these areas.

Keyword: Caries

Stainless steel clasp
These are clips made from stainless steel and are added to a partial denture which fits around a natural tooth to improve retention.

Keyword: Prosthetics

S

Standard precautions
Standard precautions have replaced the term 'universal precautions', but the same principles apply. These precautions are to protect healthcare professionals when coming into contact with blood, saliva or other body fluids. Every patient is a potential risk, even those with no obvious infectious conditions in their medical history. Standard precautions apply to all patients at all times and include policies on hand hygiene, personal protective equipment, waste disposal, clean clinical environment, decontamination of instruments and equipment and management of exposure to blood and body fluids.

Keyword: Cross-infection/health and safety

Staphylococci
Round bacteria which can be found in the mouth. The bacteria form in clumps and look similar to a bunch of grapes. These bacteria can cause boils and abscesses.

Keyword: Microbiology

Sterile gown
These come in sterile packs and are worn by operators over their normal uniform to prevent cross-infection. They need to

be put on with sterile hands and changed after use with every patient.

Keyword: Cross-infection control

Sterilisation

A process which destroys living organisms including bacteria, spores, fungi and viruses and prevents cross-infection, protecting staff and patients. Instruments should be sterilised in an autoclave with the temperature reaching 134°–137°C for three minutes.

Keyword: Cross-infection control

Sterilisation pouch

Available in different sizes to hold instruments during an autoclave cycle and to keep them sterile until opened for use. The markings on the pouch change colour indicating a successful sterilising cycle.

Keyword: Cross-infection control

Stethoscope

This instrument is used for listening to sounds in the body such as heart, lungs and blood flow. The diaphragm of the stethoscope is placed on the body and the tubing amplifies the sound through to the earpieces.

Keyword: Emergency kit

Stomach

Situated in the left side of the body under the diaphragm. Food enters this cavity of the digestive system from the oesophagus after being swallowed. Food will eventually begin to digest with the help of stomach enzymes.

Keyword: Digestion

Straight handpiece

Used during surgical procedures to remove bone. A special long shank surgical bur is attached to a motor. The handpiece also accepts acrylic burs that are used to adjust acrylic dentures.

Keyword: Handpieces and burs

Streptococcus
Bacteria which are present in the mouth and can cause infections such as tonsillitis, strep throat and scarlet fever. The bacterium is round and forms in a single line.

Keyword: Microbiology

Stroke
This is caused by the blood supply to the brain being interrupted due to a blockage of an artery or a haemorrhage near to the brain. This could result in permanent damage to the brain. Symptoms are severe headache, partial paralysis, dizziness and collapse.

Keyword: Collapse

Study models
To achieve these, upper and lower impressions are taken of the patient's teeth and are sent to the laboratory to be cast into models. They are useful to determine the occlusion of a patient before providing treatment such as crowns or bridges. They are used for orthodontic purposes to determine the best appliance and to monitor a patient who has tooth surface loss.

Keyword: Assessment

Sublingual salivary gland
Sublingual means under the tongue. This gland secretes saliva into the mouth via ducts. Saliva lubricates the mouth, initiates digestion and helps fight dental caries.

Keyword: Anatomy

Submandibular salivary gland
This salivary gland lies on the floor of the mouth near the angle of the mandible on either side and secretes saliva into the mouth under the tongue. Saliva will initiate digestion, moisten the mouth and help fight tooth decay.

Keyword: Anatomy

Sucrose
A sugar which is found naturally in fruits and vegetables. Sucrose is added to processed food as a preserve and is present in biscuits, cakes, ice-cream and many other 'junk' foods.

Keyword: Digestion

Sugar
This is a basic food carbohydrate and if taken in excessive amounts can lead to dental decay, caries, diabetes and obesity. Sugar exists as various substances in food groups such as sucrose, lactose and fructose.

Keyword: Digestion

Super floss
Recommended to patients as part of the oral health regime if they have bridges present in their mouth. The floss is made to clean the area under the pontic of the bridge where plaque will flourish in this stagnation area.

Keyword: Oral health

Superior vena cava
This large, short vein starts at the top of the chest and continues down to the right atrium of the heart. It brings blood from the head, neck and arms into the right atrium.

Keyword: Heart and circulation

Supernumerary teeth
These are extra teeth in excess of the usual number which can occur anywhere in the jaw. They are usually extracted as they can prevent the eruption of the other teeth and can cause a problem with oral hygiene.

Keyword: Anatomy

Super pluggers
Used during filling procedures to condense and pack composite material into the cavity site preventing it from sticking or discolouring the material.

Keyword: Restorations

Supra-gingival
This means just above the gum/gingival margin. Plaque and calculus can stick to this area.

Keyword: Anatomy

Surface anaesthetic
Also called topical anaesthetic. This is applied to the surface of the body only such as the gums prior to local anaesthesia being administered.

Keyword: Anaesthetic

Surface decontamination
All work surfaces should be cleared before they are disinfected. The correct detergent liquid is applied to the surface and wiped, to destroy microbes. Correct personal protection equipment should be worn and good ventilation ensured.

Keyword: Cross-infection control

Surface drape
These large covers come in sterile packs and are used to cover work surfaces to protect them and keep them sterile. They are single use only.

Keyword: Cross-infection control

Surgical bur
These latch grip burs have a long shank and attach to the straight handpiece. They are used to remove bone during a surgical procedure.

Keyword: Minor oral surgery

Surgical curette
See Spoon curette

Surgical extraction
A complex extraction which can involve the removal of soft tissue to access the roots or bone. Sometimes this is planned by the operator or a simple extraction can turn into a surgical one if the tooth breaks on removal due to a heavy filling, decay, curved roots or impaction. In some cases a gingival flap is raised to remove roots and the sutures are placed to close the incision.

Keyword: Minor oral surgery

Surgical scissors
Used during surgical procedures by the operator to cut soft tissue. They are available in different lengths, sizes and different working ends.

Keyword: Minor oral surgery

Sutures
These come in a sterile pack with a sterile needle attached. They are used to close surgical incisions and aid in healing after surgery. The sutures are made of silk and can be either dissolvable or removable.

Keyword: Minor oral surgery

Suture scissors
The blades of these scissors are designed to remove and cut sutures whilst preventing trauma to the surrounding tissues.

Keyword: Minor oral surgery

Swallowing
This process involves food or liquid entering the mouth and being chewed, mixed with saliva and being pushed to the back of the mouth. Voluntary muscles push the food into the throat, into the oesophagus towards the stomach.

Keyword: Digestion

Systemic
Describing something that affects the entire body such as a fever or high blood pressure.

Keyword:Medical condition

T

Taste buds
Located on the tongue, back of throat and the palate, these allow us to distinguish flavours. The four basic tastes are bitter, salty, sweet and sour.

Keyword: Anatomy

T ball burnisher
Referred to as a ball-ended burnisher used to smooth and polish amalgam that has just been placed in the cavity.

Keyword: Restoration

T band matrix
A single-use, metal matrix used to provide a wall during a filling procedure if the proximal surface is missing.

Keyword: Restorations

Technician
Dental laboratory technician, a professional complementary to dentistry (PCD). A qualified and trained part of the dental team who makes prosthetic and restorative appliances for patients under the instruction of the GDP.

Keyword: Dental professional

Teeth
Structures found in the upper and lower jaws used to tear and chew food, aid in speech and give the face its shape. The enamel of the tooth is the hardest substance in the body. Each tooth contains blood vessels and nerves making them respond to stimuli. The roots of the tooth fit into the jaw bone and are surrounded

by gum. Human adults have thirty two permanent teeth which erupt once the deciduous teeth are lost.

Keyword: Anatomy

Temazepam
A short-acting oral tranquilliser given one hour before treatment to relieve anxiety and promote relaxation.

Keyword: Drugs

Temperature
A degree of hot and cold of the body or of a substance. The body's normal temperature is about 37° C. When body temperature falls, we shiver, creating muscle activity which constricts blood vessels to minimise heat loss. When our temperature rises, we sweat, which dilates the blood vessels to aid in releasing excess body heat.

Keyword: Heart and circulation

Temporary bridge
Provided as a temporary cover over natural teeth and gaps from missing teeth, holding the space open preventing teeth from drifting. The impressions for the temporary bridge are taken before the extraction. It may be a while until the permanent is fitted if the extraction was recent, to allow for gums to heal and the bone to shrink.

Keyword: Prosthetic

Temporary crown
Provided as a temporary cover over a natural tooth after preparation for a permanent crown. The patient will have to wait for this lab-made prosthetic. The temporary crown will protect the natural tooth whilst waiting and will be aesthetically pleasing. It is made from a temporary material placed in an impression of the tooth, providing a natural looking tooth which will be fixed by temporary cement. The crown and cement will be easily removed, without causing destruction to the natural tooth.

Keyword: Prosthetic

Temporary restoration
Used as temporary measure until the tooth in question can be restored permanently. The material used is not as strong as permanent material. In emergency treatment, a quick setting material is used which can easily be removed at the next appointment. Sometimes a temporary restoration is provided to see if the tooth causing problems will settle down or if further investigation is needed.

Keyword: Restorations

Temporomandibular joint (TMJ)
One joint either side of the jaw, located between the condyle and the base of the skull. This joint allows the lower jaw to move. It is a synovial joint with an articulator disc allowing the rotational movement of the jaw, forwards, backwards and side to side.

Keyword: Anatomy

Tetracycline
An antibiotic drug prescribed in dentistry to patients with ulcers and periodontal disease. It can be administered as a mouthwash. It can cause staining on teeth that are still forming.

Keyword: Drugs

Therapist
A professional complementary to dentistry whose role in the team is to carry out simple fillings, pulp treatment on deciduous teeth, extractions of deciduous teeth and scaling under the instruction of the GDP.

Keyword: Dental professional

Thrush
A fungal infection also known as candidiasis which can be present orally and presents as sore, white patches in the mouth.

Keyword: Microbiology

Thyroid collar
Used in conjunction with a lead apron during x-ray taking to protect the patient from radiation. The collar is placed around the patient's neck protecting the thyroid area.

Keyword: Radiography

Tissue conditioner
A material that can be added to dentures that are rubbing on the soft tissues causing soreness. The reline material will relieve the pressure of the denture allowing tissue to heal.

Keyword: Prosthetics

Tissue dissecting forceps
A tweezers-like instrument used to retract or grasp soft tissue where suturing is taking place.

Keyword: Minor oral surgery

Tofflemire matrix retainer
This is used to hold a metal matrix band which is placed around a tooth that is being filled to provide a proximal wall. The retainer is sterilised but the band is disposed of in a sharps container.

Keyword: Restorations

Tongue
Located in the floor of the mouth attached by the lingual frenum in the mandible. It is involved in the function of swallowing, speech and mastication. It has taste buds on the base and the sides.

Keyword: Anatomy

Topical
Topical medication is applied to the surface, such as the skin or mucous membrane. Topical anaesthetic is applied to the gingiva prior to local anaesthetic being administered.

Keyword: Anaesthesia

Towel clips
Used to secure a patient's bib or any other protective clothing covering a patient. There are various types available.

Keyword: Health and safety

Trachea
Also called the windpipe, it allows the passage of air to the lungs through the throat, to the larynx, along the trachea, down the neck to the chest where it divides to form the left and right bronchi.

Keyword: Anatomy

Tranquillisers

These are drugs that have a sedative effect. They are prescribed to patients before treatment to relieve anxiety.

Keyword: Drugs

Transillumination

A strong beam of light is passed through part of the body for medical inspection. In dentistry the LED light shining through an anterior tooth will detect interproximal caries.

Keyword: Caries

Transmissible Spongiform Encephalopathies (TSEs)

This is a family of diseases that includes Creutzfeldt-Jakob disease (CJD). They are very rare but the latter stages of the disease can cause dementia which progresses rapidly.

Keyword: Pathology

Transparent film

An x-ray film can present as transparent if under-exposed or under-developed. This is why chemicals are changed regularly to dispose of weak or old solutions.

Keyword: Radiography

T

Triclosan

An essential ingredient found in toothpaste which acts as an antiseptic plaque suppressant.

Keyword: Prevention gum disease

Tricuspid valve

This valve is located in between the right ventricle and the right atrium of the heart to ensure the blood flow is only one way.

Keyword: Anatomy

Trigeminal nerve

The 5th cranial nerve. This runs from the brain stem and divides into three branches: ophthalmic division, maxillary division and mandibular division, which supplies sensation to the face, scalp, nose, teeth, lining of the mouth, upper eyelids, sinuses, front portion of the tongue and motor supply to the muscles of mastication.

Keyword: Anatomy

Trigeminal neuralgia
A disorder of the trigeminal nerve resulting in a stabbing pain which affects the cheeks, lips, gums or chin. It is usually brought on after eating, drinking, talking or even touching the face. It occurs on one side of the face and its cause is uncertain.

Keyword: Oral condition

Trimester
Term used when dividing a pregnancy into three stages of three months each.

Keyword: Pregnancy

Triple beak pliers
Used to bend and shape orthodontic archwire.

Keyword: Orthodontic

Triple trays
Single-use impression trays, loaded with impression material, designed to be used in both arches at the same time without causing discomfort to the patient.

Keyword: Impressions

Trismus
Also known as lockjaw and is caused by an involuntary muscle spasm causing the mouth to become tightly closed. Problems affecting the back teeth such as erupting wisdom teeth can cause this to happen.

Keyword: Jaw disorders

T spring
A type of spring used in orthodontic procedures added to a removable appliance to correct malocclusion.

Keyword: Orthodontic

Tuberculosis (TB)
This highly infectious disease is increasingly prevalent and is spread by airborne droplets (coughs and sneezes) or direct contact. There is evidence to prove that TB has been transmitted by dental procedures. When inhaled, the bacteria that cause the disease enter the lungs and multiply. It can spread to the lymph

nodes and other organs via the bloodstream. In most cases the body's immune system fights against the disease. A Bacillus Calmette-Guérin (BCG) vaccination is given between the ages of 10–14 years; this is a strain of the virus and has proved effective in preventing TB.

Keyword: Pathology

Tuberosity
A projection or rounded nodule existing on the areas of bone to which a muscle or tendon is attached.

Keyword: Anatomy

Tumour
This is a swelling caused by an abnormal growth of body cells in a specific area which can cause destruction to neighbouring structures. The mass can be cancerous (malignant) or non-cancerous (benign) and can spread quickly.

Keyword: Pathology

Tweed pliers
Used to bend and manipulate orthodontic archwire to form loops.

Keyword: Orthodontic

Twin block
A specialised type of removable orthodontic appliance. It is usually worn in the upper and lower jaws at the same time. Its purpose is to hold the mandible forward whilst it is still growing, keeping it in the correct class I position.

Keyword: Orthodontics

T

U

Ulcer
A sore appearing on the skin or mucous membrane caused by the destruction of soft tissue. They are usually inflamed and painful depending on the type of ulceration.

Keyword: Pathology

Ultrasonic cleaner
This piece of equipment holds a disinfectant cleaner which removes debris from instruments using sound waves. This is done before sterilisation by autoclave.

Keyword: Cross-infection control

Ultrasonic scaling tips
These tips are attached to an ultrasonic scaling unit and used to remove plaque and calculus by means of ultrasonic waves and water. It is an effective method of scaling which also removes stains from teeth.

Keyword: Periodontal

Universal curette
A periodontal hand instrument used to remove supra-gingival calculus and plaque.

Keyword: Periodontal

Universal Hobson plugger
An amalgam plugger used to pack and condense the amalgam filling into the cavity with its flat working ends.

Keyword: Restorations

Upper molar forceps
Used to extract maxillary molar teeth. They come in left and right sided and the way to determine the correct ones for use are by

placing the beak of the forceps to the buccal side, beak to cheek. Whilst looking at the patient, if the beak is pointing towards the right cheek, you have the left forceps; if the beak is pointing towards the left cheek you have the upper right forceps.

Keyword: Extractions

Upper incisor extraction forceps
These forceps are straight and are used to remove maxillary anterior teeth.

Keyword: Extractions

Upper pre-molar extraction forceps
Used to remove maxillary canines and pre-molar teeth.

Keyword: Extractions

Upper straight extraction forceps
These forceps are designed with a long thin beak to remove maxillary roots.

Keyword: Extractions

Under-cut cavity
Done purposely to aid in the retention of non-adhesive fillings. The inner surface of the cavity is wider than that of the opening of the cavity.

Keyword: Restorations

Urinary system
This body system is responsible for the excretion of urine. It is composed of the kidneys, ureter, bladder and urethra which are also concerned with the formation of urine. Blood is filtered by the kidneys to make urine which passes down the ureter into the bladder and expelled through the urethra.

Keyword: Anatomy

Urine
This liquid is produced by the kidneys when the blood is filtered removing waste and excess water. It is stored in the bladder and excreted by the body.

Keyword: Digestion

V

Vaccination
A form of immunisation whereby a particular dose of a dead micro-organism is introduced to a non-immune person by injection. This prepares the immune system for infection of that particular micro-organism in the future. Antibodies and antitoxins already present will immediately fight against the disease.

Keyword: Pathology

Vacuum autoclave
This is an item of sterilising equipment that enables instruments to be sterilised whilst sealed in pouches, within which they can then be stored until required for use, ensuring cross infection control.

Keyword: Sterilisation/cross-infection control

Vasoconstrictor
This is a constituent present in some local anaesthetics which causes the blood vessels to narrow preventing the solution from being carried away too quickly, thus prolonging the duration of the anaesthetic if the treatment required will take a while.

Keyword: Anaesthetic drug

Vein
A vessel that returns blood to the heart from various organs in the body.

Keyword: Anatomy

Veneers
A facing used to cover the buccal surface of a tooth, most commonly anterior teeth. They can be done using a composite mate-

rial by the dentist or by porcelain made in the laboratory. Impressions of the area are taken, the shade is matched and the natural tooth is prepared. Veneers are placed for aesthetic reasons if teeth are discoloured, rotated, to close a gap or to change the shape of a tooth.

Keyword: Prosthetic

Venepuncture

This is the procedure of inserting a needle into a vein to inject fluid or to draw blood. In dentistry this may be done for intravenous (IV) sedation.

Keyword: Sedation

Ventilation

A dental surgery should be well ventilated. If windows are present, then at least one should be open. If this is not possible then an extractor fan should be installed, this ventilation system should not cause risk to the public. Recycled air conditioning is not a recommended alternative. Good ventilation will reduce the risk of infection by dispersing and eliminating aerosols. Aerosol inhalation can be harmful to eyes, cause chronic coughs and bronchitis.

Keyword: Health and safety

Ventricle

A chamber in an organ. The brain has four which are filled with fluid, and the heart has two (left and right ventricles) which pump blood into the lungs or the rest of the body.

Keyword: Heart and circulation

Vertical impaction

This refers to an upright tooth that is impacted into the ramus of the lower jaw.

Keyword: Anatomy

Virus

Latin for poison or toxin. It is the smallest type of infectious agent, living in the cells of other organisms and invading them, taking them over to create copies of themselves. Antiviral drugs can be used to treat viruses as antibiotics are usually ineffective.

Keyword: Pathology

Vitality test
A simple test on a tooth can be done to determine whether a tooth is vital (alive) or non-vital (dead). A tooth that is non-vital has no blood supply to it and pulp death has occurred. Various techniques can be applied to check the tooth vitality including the use of ethyl chloride on a cotton-wool pellet. This extremely cold temperature will be felt on the tooth if it is vital. An electronic pulp tester providing an electric current to the tooth can also determine the vitality.

Keyword: Endodontic

Vital tooth
This term refers to a tooth with a living pulp contained within its inner structure. Nerves and blood vessels still supply this tooth with blood and it reacts to hot and cold stimuli.

Keyword: Endodontic

Vitamin
An essential substance required in small amount to enable the body to function normally. The main six are A, C, D, E, K and B12. There are seven grouped under the vitamin B complex. Vitamins are obtained by a balanced diet or through supplements.

Keyword: Digestion

Vocal cords
Two fibrous folds of tissue present in the larynx that vibrate at different rates to produce sound as air from the lungs passes between them.

Keyword: Respiration

Vocationally Related Qualifications (VRQ)
This is an exam governed by City & Guilds for trainees who are working towards the NVQ Oral Heath Care: Dental Nursing qualification. It contributes to the knowledge and understanding of the principles of infection control in the dental environment,

principles of oral health assessment and treatment planning, dental radiography and scientific principles in the management of plaque related diseases.

Keyword: Training

W

Wards carver
Used as a filling instrument, its flat working ends carve and shape the placed restoration in the cavity. It has sharp edges to remove excess material, make fissures like natural teeth and carves the filling so it is in the right occlusion.

Keyword: Restorations

Warfarin
An anticoagulant medication taken to help prevent blood clotting and to treat conditions such as thrombosis to prevent worsening of the disorder.

Keyword: Drugs

Warwick James elevator
Used to elevate and loosen the tooth from the periodontal ligament just before extraction, reducing trauma to the tooth tissue and bone. A patient may want an implant in the future to replace the missing tooth, so care has to be taken with the bone as this is where the implant will be seated.

Keyword: Extraction

Washer/disinfector
This is the most effective method of pre-sterilisation of instruments prior to sterilisation in the autoclave. Instruments are placed in the machine following manufacturer's instructions and put on the correct cycle. The dryer will dry the instruments after disinfected and they can then go into the autoclave.

Keyword: Cross-infection control

Wax
Various types used in dentistry to construct dentures and other prosthetics and restoratives and used to record occlusal relationships.

Keyword: Restorations/prosthetic

Wax knife
Double-ended instrument used during the construction of dentures at the bite and wax try-in stages. It is used for trimming and shaping wax.

Keyword: Prosthetic

Wedges
Can be made of wood or plastic, they are single use and their purpose is to provide support to a matrix band when placed around the tooth. This will also maintain adequate contact points between two teeth and prevent over-hanging fillings.

Keyword: Restorations

Wedjets
Used during the placement of a rubber dam sheet to ensure that it fits securely into the interproximal spaces of the tooth being isolated.

Keyword: Endodontic

Weingart pliers
Used during orthodontic procedures to guide the movement of the archwire whilst being placed in the brackets.

Keyword: Orthodontics

W

Wharton's duct
A submandibular duct connecting the submandibular salivary gland to the oral cavity. Located at the base of the tongue at the bottom of the mouth.

Keyword: Anatomy

White cells
These blood cells help defend the body against disease and infection; if it should occur, they produce protective antibodies.

Keyword: Blood

Williams periodontal probe

Used to measure the depth of the periodontal pocket around the tooth. The markings on the probe are in millimetres and measurements recorded on a special chart.

Keyword: Periodontal

Willis bite gauge

Used during the bite stage of denture construction for measuring and recording the jaw relationship, determining the height of occlusion and making sure the distance between the nose and chin is the same as the distance between the eyes and mouth.

Keyword: Prosthetic

Winter elevator

Used to elevate and loosen the tooth from the periodontal ligament just before extraction, reducing trauma to the tooth tissue and bone. This elevator blade looks like a Cryer and its handle looks like a cork screw allowing for a better grip and leverage.

Keyword: Extractions

Witness testimony

This is a piece of evidence required to be produced by an individual who is receiving training towards certification via the NVQ Oral Health Care: Dental Nursing course. The trainee nurse writes an account of a procedure witnessed by an expert, i.e. the dentist. This is used as evidence, for their portfolio, providing work-related performance criteria.

Keyword: Training

Wooden handled impression spatula

Used to mix impression material of large quantities such as alginate. Its wide metal mixing end enables the material to be mixed smoothly.

Keyword: Impressions

Wood sticks

Used to clean in between teeth (interdentally) as part of a patient's oral health routine. They look like cocktail sticks, but are not as sharp; can cause trauma to gums if used incorrectly.

Keyword: Prevention of gum disease

Work product

This is a piece of evidence required to be produced by an individual who is receiving training towards certification via the NVQ Oral Health Care: Dental Nursing course. A work product, presented in the form of non-confidential records, COSHH reports, evidence of hand washing technique, is used as evidence of knowledge and understanding of specific principles, and is entered into the trainee's portfolio.

Keyword: Training

W

X

Xerostomia

This is the medical term for a dry mouth due to lack of saliva. This causes problems with speech and eating and can lead to halitosis, gum disease and an increase of dental caries.

Keyword: Digestion/Oral Disease

X-rays

Also called radiographs, taken during the diagnosis of treatment. The image of the bone, organ or tissue is formed by electromagnetic radiation of a short wave-length and high energy, producing the image onto a film or screen for viewing.

Keyword: Radiography

X-ray developer

A fluid used in the first stage of processing an x-ray. Used during automatic and manual developing. The film stays in the developing solution until the image has been developed, then the film is immersed in water to remove the excess fluid and placed in fixer fluid.

Keyword: Radiography

X-ray fixer

A fluid used in the second stage of processing an x-ray. After the film has been developed and immersed in water to remove excess developer solution, the image will need to be fixed to create a permanent image which is not sensitive to light; it will need to be immersed in water again and dried. Used during automatic and manual developing.

Keyword: Radiography

X-ray viewer

A portable piece of equipment with a built in light source and magnifier allowing an x-ray to be mounted on and viewed.

Keyword: Radiography

X

Z

Zinc oxide-eugenol cement
Used as a temporary restoration for emergency procedures. It is also used as a lining in deep cavities as a sedative dressing. The zinc oxide powder and eugenol (oil of cloves) are mixed together on a glass slab to the required amount and consistency.

Keyword: Restorations

Zinc phosphate cement
This zinc oxide powder and phosphoric acid liquid are mixed together on a glass slab to the required amount and consistency. The cement is used for temporary restorations, linings and cement for fixing crowns.

Keyword: Restorations

Zinc polycarboxylate cement
A zinc oxide and polyacrylic acid powder is mixed with sterile water on a glass slab with a metal spatula and is used as a temporary restoration, luting cement and lining during endodontic treatment.

Keyword: Restorations

Zoning
This is the separating areas of the surgery into a dirty zone and a clean zone to prevent cross-infection and contamination

Keyword: Cross-infection

Z spring
A type of spring used on an orthodontic removable appliance to correct malocclusion.

Keyword: Orthodontics

Zygomatic arch

This is the bone we refer to as the cheek bone on either side of the skull/temporal bone.

Keyword: Anatomy

Z

Part 2

Appendices and Charts

Chart One

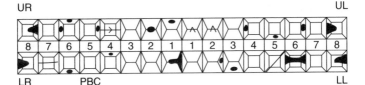

Upper right 8:- MO amalgam present

Upper right 7:- Sound tooth

Upper right 6:- Distal and buccal fillings present

Upper right 5:- Mesial filling present

Upper right 4:- Tooth missing space closed

Upper right 3:- Sound tooth

Upper right 2:- Incisal filling present

Upper right 1:- Labial filling present

Lower right 8:- DO filling present

Lower right 7:- Missing

Lower right 6:- Buccal filling present

Upper left 1:- Missing/partial denture

Upper left 2:- Missing/partial denture

Upper left 3:- Sound tooth

Upper left 4:- Mesial filling present

Upper left 5:- Palatal filling present

Upper left 6:- Distal filling present

Upper left 7:- Sound tooth

Upper left 8:- MO filling present

Lower left 1:- Sound tooth

Lower left 2:- Distal filling present

Lower left 3:- Labial filling present

Lower right 5:- Porcelain bonded crown present

Lower right 4:- Lingual filling present

Lower right 3:- Sound tooth

Lower right 2:- Sound tooth

Lower right 1:- Mesial incisal filling present

Lower left 4:- Sound tooth

Lower left 5:- To be extracted

Lower left 6:- MOD filling present

Lower left 7:- Sound tooth

Lower left 8:- DO filling present

Chart Two

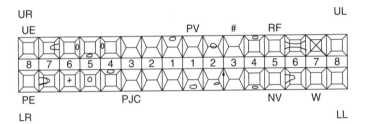

Upper right 8:- Un-erupted tooth

Upper right 7:- MO cavity

Upper right 6:- Mesial cavity

Upper right 5:- Palatal cavity

Upper right 4:- Distal cavity

Upper right 3:- Sound tooth

Upper right 2:- Sound tooth

Upper right 1:- Labial cavity

Lower right 8:- Partially erupted

Lower right 7:- DO cavity

Lower right 6:- Retained root

Lower right 5:- Occlusal cavity

Lower right 4:- Lingual cavity

Upper left 1:- Porcelain veneer present

Upper left 2:- Incisal cavity

Upper left 3:- Has a fracture

Upper left 4:- Buccal cavity

Upper left 5:- Root filling present

Upper left 6:- MOD cavity

Upper left 7:- Recently extracted

Upper left 8:- Sound tooth

Lower left 1:- Labial cavity

Lower left 2:- Sound tooth

Lower left 3:- Sound tooth

Lower left 4:- Buccal cavity

Lower left 5:- Non vital

Lower right 3:- Porcelain
jacket crown present
Lower right 2:- Sound tooth
Lower right 1:- Sound tooth

Lower left 6:- MO cavity

Lower left 7:- Watch
Lower left 8:- Sound tooth

FDI Chart

UR8	UR7	UR6	UR5	UR4	UR3	UR2	UR1	UL1	UL2	UL3	UL4	UL5	UL6	UL7	UL8
LR8	LR7	LR6	LR5	LR4	LR3	LR2	LR1	LL1	LL2	LL3	LL4	LL5	LL6	LL7	LL8

FDI two-digit system for permanent teeth

quadrant 1	quadrant 2
quadrant 4	quadrant 3

18	17	16	15	14	13	12	11	21	22	23	24	25	26	27	28
48	47	46	45	44	43	42	41	31	32	33	34	35	36	37	38

The quadrant symbol is replaced by a number, e.g. the upper right quadrant now becomes quadrant 1.

The quadrant number forms the first digit and the second digit is the tooth number, e.g. UR8 now becomes 18; UL 8 now becomes 28, and so on.

The chart is read starting from the upper right side to the upper left and lower left to the lower right side. The upper right E now becomes 55, the lower left E now becomes 75.

E	D	C	B	A	A	B	C	D	E
E	D	C	B	A	A	B	C	D	E

FDI two-digit system for deciduous teeth

quadrant 5	quadrant 6
quadrant 8	quadrant 7

55	54	53	52	51	61	62	63	64	65
85	84	83	82	81	71	72	73	74	75

Abbreviations and Definitions

PROFESSIONAL BODIES, QUALIFICATIONS ETC

Abbreviation	Definition
BADN	British Association of Dental Nurses
BDS	Bachelor of Dental Surgery
CPD	Continuing Professional Development
DDR	Diploma in Dental Radiography
DGDP	Diploma in General Dental Practice
DNSTAB	Dental Nurses Standards & Training Advisory Board
DPB	Dental Practice Board
DRO	Dental Reference Officer
EDH	Enrolled Dental Hygienist
EDT	Enrolled Dental Therapist
FDI	International Dental Federation
GDC	General Dental Council
GDP	General Dental Practitioner
GP	General Practitioner
M Paed Dent	Membership in Paediatric Dentistry
MDS	Master of Dental Surgery
MFDS	Membership of the Faculty of Dental Surgery
MGDP	Membership in General Dental Practice
MGDS	Member in General Dental Surgery
MOrth	Member in Orthodontics
MRD	Member in Restorative Dentistry
MSc	Master of Science
NEBDN	National Examining Board of Dental Nurses

NHS	National Health Service
NHS BAS	National Health Service Business Advisory Service
NRPB	National Radiological Protection Board
NVQ	National Vocational Qualification
PCD	Professional Complementary to Dentistry
PCT	Primary Care Trust
RDT	Registered Dental Technician
RPA	Radiation Protection Advisor
RPS	Radiation Protection Supervisor

MATERIALS

Abbreviation	Definition
CO_2	Carbon Dioxide
ETB	Electric Toothbrush
GP	Gutta-Percha
H_2O	Water
LA	Local Anaesthetic
M/W	Mouth Wash
N_2O	Nitrous Oxide
O_2	Oxygen
PenV	Penicillin
T/P	Toothpaste
TB	Toothbrush
ZOE	Zinc Oxide & Eugenol Cement

ORAL LOCATIONS

Abbreviation	Definition
B	Buccal
D	Distal
DIV	Division
I	Inciscal
L	Lingual
LHS	Left Hand Side
LL	Lower Left
LLQ	Lower Left Quadrant
LR	Lower Right
LRQ	Lower Right Quadrant

M	Mesial
MM	Muscles of Mastication
O	Occlusal
P	Palatal
RHS	Right Hand Side
TMJ	Temporo-Mandibular Joint
UL	Upper Left
ULQ	Upper Left Quadrant
UR	Upper Right
URQ	Upper Right Quadrant
X Bite	Cross Bite
↑	Upper
↓	Lower

APPOINTMENT MANAGEMENT

Abbreviation	Definition
1/52, 2/52, 3/52	1 Week, 2 Weeks, 3 Weeks, etc
12/12	12 Months
3/12	3 Months
6/12	6 Months
CICF	Card In Current File
DNA	Did Not Attend
DNR	Did Not Return
FTA	Failed To Attend
FTR	Failed To Return
MA	Missed Appointment
OP	Old Patient
PCO	Patient Complaining Of
R/V	Review
TC	Treatment Complete
TCA	To Come Again

DIAGNOSIS

Abbreviation	Definition
#	Fracture
ANUG	Acute Necrotising Ulcerative Gingivitis
BOP	Bleeding On Probing
DMF	Decayed, Missing, Filled

IOTN	Index of Orthodontic Treatment Need
PE	Partially Erupted
PN	Pain
TA	Toothache
TTP	Tender To Percussion
UE	Unerupted

TREATMENT

Abbreviation	Definition
-/F	Full Lower Denture
-/P	Partial Lower Denture
A/F	Amalgam Filling
AMG	Amalgam
B/F	Bridge Fit
B/P	Bridge Preparation
BA	Bridge Abutment
BP	Bridge Pontic
BPE	Basic Periodontal Exam
BSS	Braided Silk Suture
BW	Bite Wing X-Rays
C/F	Crown Fit
C/P	Crown Preparation
CM	Composite Filling
DPT	Dental Panoramic Tomograph
F/-	Full Upper Denture
F/F	Full Upper & Lower Denture
F/S	Fissure Sealant
FGC	Full Gold Crown
FVC	Full Veneer Crown
GI	Gold Inlay
GIC	Glass Ionomer Cement
OHI	Oral Hygiene Instruction
OPG	Panoral Orthopantomograph
P/-	Partial Upper Denture
PA	Periapical X-Rays
PAL	Probing Attachment Loss
PBC	Porcelain Bonded Crown
PC	Post Crown

PJC	Porcelain Jacket Crown
POIG	Post Operative Instructions Given
PPD	Probing Pocket Depth
PV	Porcelain Veneer
RCT	Root Canal Treatment
REF	Referral
ROS	Removal Of Suture
S/P	Scale & Polish
TM	Temporary Filling
TMT	Treatment
UDA	Unit of Dental Activity
V/F	Veneer Fit
V/P	Veneer Preparation
XGA	Extraction Under General Anaesthetic
XLA	Extraction Under Local Anaesthetic

GENERAL

Abbreviation	Definition
AIDS	Acquired Immune Deficiency Syndrome
BNF	British National Formulary
CS	Conscious Sedation
DPF	Dental Practitioners Formulary
DPT	Dental Panoramic Tomograph
GA	General Anaesthesia
HBV	Hepatitis B Virus
HCV	Hepatitis C Virus
HIV	Human Immunodeficiency Virus
IV	Intravenous
MG	Milligrams
MH	Medical History
MTB	Manual Toothbrush
NME	Non-Milk Extrinsic (Sugar)
NP	New Patient
NSAID	Non-Steroidal Anti-Inflammatory Drug
O/E	On Examination
OH	Oral Hygiene
PT	Patient

| R/X | Prescription |
| RA | Relative Analgesia |

HEALTH & SAFETY AND FIRST AID

Abbreviation	Definition
ABC	Airway, Breathing, Circulation
ALARA	As Low As Reasonably Achievable
ALS	Advanced Life Support
BLS	Basic Life Support
BP	Blood Pressure
COSHH	Control Of Substances Hazardous to Health
CPR	Cardio Pulmonary Resuscitation
DRABC	Dangers Responsiveness Airway Breathing Circulation
EAV	Expired Air Ventilation
ECC	External Cardiac Compression
ECG	Electro Cardio Gram
IRR	Ionising Radiation Regulations
RIDDOR	Reporting of Injuries, Diseases & Dangerous Occurrences Regulations

Training and Accreditation

In order to become a dental nurse, candidates need to gain qualification in one of the following GDC approved awards:

CITY & GUILDS LEVEL 3 NVQ IN ORAL HEALTH CARE:
DENTAL NURSING (3231-23/83)
This NVQ is aimed at dental nurses who, along with other members of the dental team, work in a variety of settings including general dental practices, the community dental service, dental and general hospitals and the armed services. The learner's role would range from reception duties and practice management to maintaining materials and equipment, cross-infection control, support for the patient and the dentist during clinical procedures and oral health education.

This level 3 qualification is aimed at people who provide direct chairside work, patient care and support during a range of dental treatments.

This qualification has been especially designed with the support of the National Examination Board for Dental Nurses (NEBDN) to meet the needs of dental nurses.

AND

CITY & GUILDS LEVEL 3 AWARD IN DENTAL NURSING (7393-01)
The new level 3 VRQ in Dental Nursing allows learners to develop the knowledge required for full-time employment and/or career progression in the dental sector. It also provides valuable accreditation of knowledge and understanding towards the related level 3 NVQ in Dental Nursing.

OR

NEBDN NATIONAL CERTIFICATE IN DENTAL NURSING
Dental nurses support other members of the oral health care team across the full range of dental treatment. Consequently, the scope of the syllabus for dental nursing is very wide.

There is open access to the examination for any person working as a dental nurse. However, candidates who are successful will not be awarded the qualification until completion of 24 months full-time (or part-time equivalent) practical experience as a dental nurse. Those not having completed 24 months at the date of the examination will receive a form with their examination result to be returned to NEBDN on completion of the required experience. The National Certificate Examination consists of five sections and candidates are required to pass all sections. However, a borderline failure in one section can be compensated by a good pass in another section.

School of Professionals Complementary to Dentistry (Portsmouth University), CertHE in Dental Nursing
This is a 15-month, full-time course, starting in October each year, enabling students to attain an academic award as well as professional registration as a qualified dental nurse.

Key academic and clinical topics covered include:

- Health, safety and infection control procedures
- General and oral anatomy and physiology
- Human and oral diseases (pathology, microbiology)
- Preparation and maintenance of instruments, materials and equipment necessary for dental procedures
- Methods of assisting the operator (e.g. dentist, dental therapist) during all patient treatment requirements (e.g. filling, crowns, bridges, extraction of teeth, surgical procedures, orthodontics)
- Patient management techniques
- Preventative dentistry
- Dental public health
- Law and ethics

- Reflective practice and professionalism
- Processing, mounting and quality assurance techniques associated with taking dental radiographs.

Places on the course are limited, and demand is usually high; an interview process determines candidate suitability based on the following criteria and qualifications:

- A genuine interest in the care and treatment of patients as part of the dental team
- A period of work placement in dental practice
- Team working ability
- Excellent verbal and written communication skills
- Some IT experience
- A high level of commitment due to the intensive nature of this academic and clinical programme
- One science based A2 award/2 passes at AS level or equivalent
- 4 GCSEs (grades A-C), or equivalent, including one science-based subject
- Mature entry (over 21 years of age) via the accreditation of prior learning (assessed on application).

Professional Progression Routes

DENTAL HYGIENIST

Before you can work as a dental hygienist, you need to take a General Dental Council (GDC) approved course. You can qualify by taking:

A Diploma in Dental Hygiene or Dental Hygiene and Dental Therapy (two years full-time)

OR

A BSc in Oral Health Science or Dental Therapy and Dental Hygiene.

To get onto either course, you will usually need:

Five GCSEs (A-C), including English and a biological science

AND

Two A levels or equivalent qualifications or a recognised dental nurse qualification.

DENTAL THERAPIST

To become a dental therapist you need to take a General Dental Council (GDC) approved course, such as:

A diploma in dental therapy (often combined with a diploma in dental hygiene)

OR

A degree in oral health sciences or dental therapy and dental hygiene.

DENTAL TECHNICIAN

To get on to an approved dental technology course you are likely to need:

BTEC national diploma – four GCSEs (A-C) including English, mathematics and a science

Foundation degree – one A level, as well as four GCSEs

Degree – five GCSEs (A-C) plus two or three A levels.

SPECIALIST DENTAL NURSING

The **Certificate in Dental Sedation Nursing** is a qualification suitable for dental nurses who assist in the surgery during routine conscious sedation. This examination is only suitable for candidates engaged in this type of work on a regular basis as the completion of a Portfolio of Experience, including a log sheet, is a requirement for the examination.

In order to qualify for the award, a dental nurse must:

a) Hold a registerable qualification
b) Be on the current Voluntary National Register of Dental Nurses
c) Have the support of their dentist/sedationist who will be required to validate the workplace activities for the Portfolio of Experienced Implant co-ordinator.

The National Examining Board for Dental Nurses (NEBDN) holds an examination for a **Certificate in Oral Health Education**. This tests the practical skills and theoretical background necessary for the provision of health education in dental practice in a one to one situation or in small groups.

In order to qualify for entry to the examination, a dental nurse must:

a) Hold a registrable qualification
b) Be on the current Voluntary National Register of Dental Nurses
c) Have the agreement of a dentist to act as supervisor before their application for the examination can be accepted.

The **Certificate in Orthodontic Nursing** is a qualification suitable for dental nurses who assist in orthodontic procedures.

The qualification is only available through approved training centres. Students will be required to attend a programme of theoretical instruction and also compile evidence of practical competence through a Portfolio of Experience.

In order to qualify for the award, a dental nurse must:

a) Hold a registrable qualification
b) Be on the current Voluntary National Register of Dental Nurses
c) Have the support of their employer who will be required to allow time and access for training at an approved training centre
d) Validate the workplace activities for the Portfolio of Experience.

The **Certificate in Dental Radiography for Dental Nurses** is a qualification suitable for dental nurses who may act as an operator under the Ionising Radiation (Medical Exposure) Regulations (IR(ME)R) 2000.

In order to qualify for the award, a dental nurse must:

a) Have a registerable dental nurse qualification
b) Enrol with NEBDN
c) Have the support of their supervisor/trainer, normally their employing GDP who will sign the "Completion of Training Form".

NVQ ASSESSOR/TUTOR

The A1 Assessors Award course is to prepare people to assess National Vocational Qualifications in the workplace, providing you have the experience and knowledge in the occupational area you are going to assess. In order to teach the occupational area you will need to achieve one of the following qualifications:

Award in Preparing to Teach in the Lifelong Learning Sector (PTLLS)
Certificate in teaching in the Life Long Learning Sector (CTTLS)
Diploma in Teaching in the Life Long Learning Sector-Level 5 (DTLLS)

Compulsory General Dental Council (GDC) Registration for Dental Care Professionals (DCPs)

GDC registration licenses dental professionals to work in the UK; *all* dental nurses and dental technicians *must* be registered as of 31 July 2008. The GDC is the regulatory body of the dental profession. Its powers, awarded by parliament, currently cover all registered members of the Dental Care Professionals team (dentists, hygienists, nurses, technicians, etc.), protecting patients by;

- Keeping up-to-date lists of properly qualified dentists, dental hygienists and dental therapists
- Setting high standards of dental practice and conduct
- Maintaining high standards of dental education
- Requiring dentists to take part in continuing professional development to keep their knowledge and skills up-to-date
- Taking action if there is doubt about whether a dental professional should be allowed to continue practising dentistry.

Registration requires an individual to demonstrate that they meet the relevant standards for entry on the DCP register, and to make payment accordingly. Once registered, you become professionally accountable for your conduct and fitness to practise; in real terms, if a complaint is made against a registered member, the GDC will investigate and action can be taken.

Before 31 July 2008, dental nurses without a formal qualification, but who had been employed full time in practice for four of the last eight years, were eligible for entry to the register. However, annual re-registration (from 2009) will only be available to those nurses without a qualification who are currently in training for a GDC accredited award (table 1).

From 31 July 2008, trainee dental nurses working in practice, with less than four years' experience, must be enrolled on a recognised training course leading to qualification. You do not need to be registered with the GDC during this time; upon qualification, registration will then be mandatory for you to continue practising.

From 31 July 2008, in order to register, all dental nurses must hold one of qualifications from the following table.

Table 1 Qualifications and awarding bodies

Qualification	Awarding Body
National Certificate in Dental Nursing	National Examining Board for Dental Nurses (NEBDN)
NVQ Level 3 in Oral Healthcare	City & Guilds/NEBDN
SVQ Level 3 in Oral Healthcare	Scottish Qualifications Authority/NEBDN
Certificate of Proficiency in Dental Nursing	Dental Hospital recognised by Association of Dental Hospitals
Certificate of Higher Education in Dental Nursing	The University of Portsmouth

PROFESSIONAL INDEMNITY INSURANCE

Current GDC guidelines, as of March 2008, strongly suggest that all dental professionals protect themselves in respect of potential compensation claims by patients with a suitable indemnity insurance policy. Examples of reasons for patient claims against a registered nurse include:

- committing an act of malpractice or negligence
- providing wrongful advice
- breaching confidentiality.

Various schemes are available, either through your employer (check your terms of employment), through private insurance companies that specialise in medical/dental policies (Dental Protection), or through the BADN, who operate a GDC-compliant scheme for all full members.

Continuing Professional Development (CPD) and CPD Form

Continuing Professional Development is the term applied to any training courses, seminars, study, reading or other activities that you do to further your knowledge and experience in your profession.

There are two types of CPD: verifiable and general. Verifiable CPD is any activity which has specific educational aims, objectives and outcomes, documentary proof (certificate) of attendance, as well as the facility to provide post-course evaluation. General CPD covers all other activities that are self-directed in the area of personal professional development, such as reading journals and private study.

A CPD cycle covers a five-year period during registration, and requires that you complete 150 hours CPD in total within this period, a minimum of 50 hours of which needs to be verifiable. These 50 hours also need to include the following core subjects:

- medical emergencies (10 hours per cycle)
- disinfection and decontamination (5 hours per cycle)
- radiography and radiation protection (5 hours per cycle).

Continuing Professional Development (CPD)

Five Year Cycle (150hrs) Activity Record Sheet, with core subject reminder

Blackwell Publishing

Name:	Title: Miss/Mrs/Ms/Mr/Dr/Other
GDC Reg. No:	Medical Emergencies (10hrs per cycle)
	Disinfection & Decontamination (5hrs per cycle)
	Radiography & Radiation Protection (5hrs per cycle)

Course/Activity Title	Date of Course	Venue	Hours	Provider	Verifiable?	Comments
			Total Hours			

Professional Bodies, Publications and Useful Websites

British Association of Dental Nurses
PO Box 4
Room 200
Hillhouse International
  Business Centre
Thornton-Cleveleys
FY5 4QD
Tel: 01253 338 360
Fax: 01253 773 266
Website: www.badn.org.uk
Email: admin@badn.org.uk
  (for general enquiries)

General Dental Council
37 Wimpole Street
London
W1G 8DQ
Tel: 0845 222 4141
Fax: 020 7224 3294
Website: www.gdc-uk.org
Email: ces@gdc-uk.org

National Examining Board for Dental Nurses
110 London Street
Fleetwood
Lancashire
FY7 6EU
Tel: 01253 778 417
Email: info@nebdn.org
Website: www.nebdn.org.uk

City & Guilds
1 Giltspur Street
London
EC1A 9DD
Tel: 020 7294 2800
Fax: 020 7294 2400
Website: www.city-and-guilds.co.uk
Email: learnersupport@cityandguilds.com

British Dental Association
64 Wimpole Street
London
W1G 8YS
Tel: 020 7935 0875
Fax: 020 7487 5232
Website: www.bda.org
Email: enquiries@bda.org

PUBLICATIONS

Title	Author	ISBN
Levison's Textbook for Dental Nurses	Carole Hollins	9781405175579
NVQs for Dental Nurses	Carole Hollins	9781405105286
Basic Guide to Dental Instruments	Carmen Scheller	9781405133791
Handbook for Dental Nurses	Jane Bonehill, Clare Roberts, Diana Wincott	9781405128032
Radiography and Radiology for Dental Nurses	Eric Whaites	9780443102134
The British Dental Nurses Journal	Quarterly magazine from BADN	
Vital	Quarterly magazine from the BDA, supplementary to BDJ	
British Dental Journal	Fortnightly magazine from the BDA	
Dental Nursing Magazine	www.dental-nursing.co.uk	

USEFUL WEBSITES

Royal Air Force Dental Careers
www.raf.mod.uk
Royal Army Dental Careers
www.army.mod.uk
Dental Technologists Association
www.dta-uk.org
British Association of Dental Therapists
www.badt.org.uk
Portsmouth University (School of Professionals Complementary to Dentistry)
www.port.ac.uk
Tempdent Dental Agency
www.tempdent.co.uk
DenMed Training & Consultancy
www.denmed-uk.com
Dental Protection
www.dentalprotection.org

Royal Navy Dental Careers
www.royalnavy.mod.uk

NHS Careers
www.nhscareers.nhs.uk

MediCruit Dental Recruitment
www.medi-cruit.co.uk

British Dental Health Foundation
www.dentalhealth.org.uk

Smile-On.com
www.smile-on.com
Dentaid
www.dentaid.org